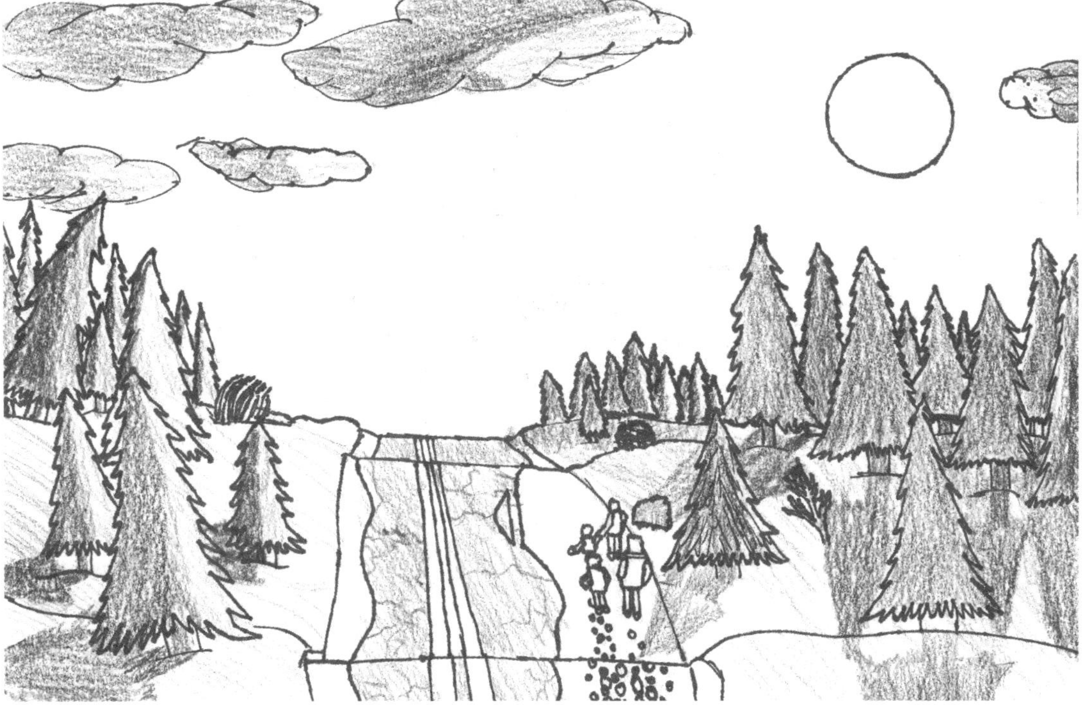

ᕈᐢ ᓯᐧᐋᓗ ᐅᑎᐹᒋᒧᐧᐃᓐ ᒋᓵᓰᐲᐦᒡ ᐅᐦᒌᐤ

ᐧᕉᐢ ᓯᐧᐋᐧᓛ ᐅᑎᐹᒋᒧᐧᐃᓐ, ᒋᓴᓰᐲᐅᐄᓅ

L’histoire de Rose Swallow de Chisasibi

The Story of Rose Swallow of Chisasibi

Told by Rose Swallow
Written by Ruth DyckFehderau
Translated into Northern East Cree by Luci Bobbish-Salt
Translated into Southern East Cree by Louise Blacksmith
Translated into French by Valérie Duro

ᒥᔪᐲᒫᑎᓰᐅᓐ ᐊᓅᓅᑭᒋᐦᒑᑭᓅᒻ
CONSEIL CRI DE LA SANTÉ ET DES SERVICES SOCIAUX DE LA BAIE JAMES
CREE BOARD OF HEALTH AND SOCIAL SERVICES OF JAMES BAY

Funding for this publication was provided in part by Health Canada. The opinions expressed in this publication are those of the storyteller and do not necessarily reflect the official views of Health Canada or of the Cree Board of Health and Social Services of James Bay.

Some names and details in this book may have been changed for the purpose of protecting identities. Any similarities between these changed names or details and real persons, living or dead, is not intended.

First printing, 2020. Printed and bound in Canada by Houghton Boston Printers, Saskatoon, Saskatchewan. Distributed by Wilfrid Laurier University Press / wlupress.wlu.ca

Set in Verdana font, chosen for its readability. Printed on paper that is Forest Stewardship Council-certified with post-consumer recycled fibres, and that is acid- and chlorine-free.

Cover design by Nicole Ritzer, based on an original design by Cameron Mosimann. Photograph of Mistissini burnt forest (reversed) taken by David DyckFehderau. Title page illustration by Jarred Voyageur of Mikw Chiyâm Arts Concentration Program, Voyageur Memorial High School, Mistissini, QC.

Published by Cree Board of Health and Social Services of James Bay
Contact: Paul Linton, 168 Main St, Mistissini, QC, Canada, G0W 1C0 / (418) 923-3355
creehealth.org / sweetbloods.org

Library and Archives Canada Cataloguing in Publication

Title: Rus siwaalu utipaachimuwin chisaasiipiihch uhchiiu = Raas siwaalwaa utipaachimuwin, chisesiipiiuiinuu = L'histoire de Rose Swallow de Chisasibi = The story of Rose Swallow of Chisasibi / story by Rose Swallow ; translator Northern East Cree, Luci Bobbish-Salt ; translator Southern East Cree, Louise Blacksmith ; translator French Valérie Duro ; writer, Ruth DyckFehderau.

Other titles: Raas siwaalwaa utipaachimuwin, chisesiipiiuiinuu | Histoire de Rose Swallow de Chisasibi | Story of Rose Swallow of Chisasibi

Names: DyckFehderau, Ruth, author. | DyckFehderau, Ruth, 1967- Story of Rose Swallow of Chisasibi. | DyckFehderau, Ruth, 1967- Story of Rose Swallow of Chisasibi. Cree. | DyckFehderau, Ruth, 1967- Story of Rose Swallow of Chisasibi. French. | Cree Board of Health and Social Services of James Bay, issuing body.

Description: Cree title romanized. | "This is a four-language translation of a single story from The Sweet Bloods of Eeyou Istchee: Stories of Diabetes and the James Bay Cree. (Sweet Bloods contains 26 stories.)" | Text in Northern East Cree, Southern East Cree, French, and English.

Identifiers: Canadiana 20200402528E | ISBN 9781989796047 (softcover)

Subjects: LCSH: Swallow, Rose—Health. | LCSH: Diabetics—Cree Nation of Chisasibi—Biography. | LCGFT: Biographies.

Classification: LCC RC660 .D96 2020 | DDC 362.1964/620092—dc23

Catalogage avant publication de Bibliothèque et Archives Canada
Titre: Rus siwaalu utipaachimuwin chisaasiipiihch uhchiiu = Raas siwaalwaa utipaachimuwin, chisesiipiiuiinuu = L'histoire de Rose Swallow de Chisasibi = The story of Rose Swallow of Chisasibi / story by Rose Swallow ; translator Northern East Cree, Luci Bobbish-Salt ; translator Southern East Cree, Louise Blacksmith ; translator French Valérie Duro ; writer, Ruth DyckFehderau.
Autres titres: Raas siwaalwaa utipaachimuwin, chisesiipiiuiinuu | Histoire de Rose Swallow de Chisasibi | Story of Rose Swallow of Chisasibi
Noms: DyckFehderau, Ruth, 1967- auteur. | DyckFehderau, Ruth, 1967- Story of Rose Swallow of Chisasibi. | DyckFehderau, Ruth, 1967- Story of Rose Swallow of Chisasibi. Cree. | DyckFehderau, Ruth, 1967- Story of Rose Swallow of Chisasibi. Français. | Conseil Cri de la santé et des services sociaux de la Baie-James, organisme de publication.
Description: Titre cri romanisé. | Publiée antérieurement dans : The Sweet Bloods of Eeyou Istchee: Stories of Diabetes and the James Bay Cree. | Texte en cri de l'Est du nord, en cri de l'Est du sud, en français et en anglais.
Identifiants: Canadiana 20200402528F | ISBN 9781989796047 (couverture souple)
Vedettes-matière: RVM: Swallow, Rose—Santé. | RVM: Diabétiques—Cree Nation of Chisasibi—Biographies. | RVMGF: Biographies.
Classification: LCC RC660 .D96 2020 | CDD 362.1964/620092—dc23

ᐋᔥᒄ ᐋᐦ ᒌᐦ ᐊᐧᐋᔑᔒᐧᐃᐨ ᕈᔅ, ᐋᔥᒄ ᓂᒧ ᐅᐦᒋ ᐲᐦᒋᑳᐤ ᒋᔅᑯᑎᒫᑑᑭᒥᑯᐦᒡ, ᑳ ᒌ ᐧᐄᒑᐧᐋᐨ ᐅᒥᔓᒻᐦ ᐋᐦ ᒋᔥᒋᐱᔨᔨᒡᐦ ᐊᑎᒻᐦ ᐋᐦ ᐋᐱᒋᐦᐋᔨᒡᐦ ᓈᑖᐦ ᐧᐄᓂᐹᑯᐦᒡ ᑳ ᒌ ᐄᔅᐱᔨᔨᒡ ᑭᔮᐦ ᐊᓂᑖᐦ ᐋᑎᔥᑎᐧᑳᔮᔨᒡ ᒋᓵᓲᐲᔨᐤ ᐋᐦ ᓈᑎᐦᐄᐹᒡ, ᐅᒧᔓᒻᐦ ᐋᐦ ᒌᐦ ᐱᐧᑳᐦᐄᐹᔨᒡᐦ᙮ ᐊᓂᑖᐦ ᐲᐦᒡ ᐅᑖᐹᓈᔅᑯᐦᒡ ᐋᑯᑖᐦ ᑳ ᒌ ᐊᐱᐨ ᐧᐄᔨ ᕈᔅ, ᓈᔥᒡ ᐋᐦ ᒋᔑᐧᐋᔨᐦᑎᒥᔨᒡᐦ ᐋᐦ ᐱᒥᐱᐦᑖᔨᒡᐦ ᐅᑖᒥᐧᐋᐤᐦ ᐊᓂᑎᐦ ᐅᐦᐱᒫ ᐋᐦ ᐱᒦᐱᐦᑖᔨᒡᐦ ᐅᒧᔓᒻᐦ᙮ ᓂᔮᓂᑯᑑᓐᐦ ᐋᐦ ᑎᐦᑯᒋᐦᐱᔨᐦᐧᐃᔨᒡᐦ ᐅᑖᐹᓈᔅᑯᐦᒡ ᐅᒧᔓᒻᐦ ᐧᐋᔨᐱᔥᒌᔥ ᐋᐦ ᐋᔨᐧᐋᔑᔨᒡᐦ᙮

“ᐧᐋᐱᒥᒡ ᒫ,” ᐄᑎᑰ ᐅᒧᔓᒻᐦ, “ᐋᔥᐱᔑ ᑭᒑᐦᑖᐧᐋᔨᐦᑎᐦᒡᐦ ᐊᑎᒧᒡ᙮ ᒋᔅᒑᔨᐦᑎᒧᔅ ᐧᐋᔥ ᐊᓂᑖᐦ ᐋᐦ ᐱᐱᑭᑎᓂᔨᒡ ᐋᑯᐦ ᓂᒥ ᐄᔅᐱᐦᑖᐧᐃᒡ ᐊᓂᑖᐦ᙮ ᐋᑯᑎᐦ ᒫᒃ ᓈᑖᐦ ᐃᐦᐄᐲᒡ ᐋᐦ ᐄᐦᑖᒡ ᐋᑯᑖᐦ ᒑ ᒌᐦ ᐄᔅᐱᔨᔨᒄᐦ, ᐊᓂᑖᐦ ᐋᐦ ᒋᔑᒋᐧᐃᒡᐦ ᑭᔮᐦ ᐊᑎᑎᐤ ᐋᐦ ᒫᔮᑎᐦᒡ, ᐋᔪᐧᐃᒄ ᐧᐄᔨᐧᐋᐤ ᐊᔥᑖᒥᓅᒡ ᐋᐦ ᒋᔅᒑᔨᑎᐦᒡᐦ ᐊᓂᑖᐦ ᓈᐦᐋᐤ ᒑ ᐄᔅᐱᐦᐄᑐᒡ᙮”

ᑖᐹ ᐅᐦᒋ ᐧᐄᐦ ᐃᔮᐧᐃᔮᐤ ᐊᓂᔮᐦ ᐊᑎᒻᐦ, ᐋᑯᐦ ᒦᓐ ᑳ ᒌ ᐋᒥᐱᔨᐦᐅᐨ ᒦᓐ ᒑ ᐱᒥᐱᐦᑖᐨ ᐋᐦ ᑎᐦᑯᓈᐨ ᐊᓂᔮᐦ ᐅᑖᐹᓈᔅᒄᐦ᙮

ᐧᐋᑎᐦᑖᐧᑖᐤᐦ ᐃᐦᐄᐲᐦ, ᑳ ᒌ ᐋᒦᐨ ᐊᓂᑎᐦ ᐅᐦᒋ ᐅᑖᐹᓈᔅᑯᐦᒡ ᕈᔅ ᑭᔮᐦ ᑳ ᒌ ᐊᔨᐧᐋᔑᒡ

ᑳ ᐊᐱᔒᔒᐨ ᐧᕌᔅ ᐁᔅᒄ ᐁᑳ ᐅᐦᒋ ᐲᐦᒉᐨ ᒋᔅᑯᑕᒫᒉᐅᑲᒥᑯᔫ ᐅᒧᔔᒻ ᒌ ᐧᐄᒉᐧᐁᐤ ᐁ ᓇᑕᐦᐄᐯᔨᒡ᙮ ᒌ ᒌᔔᐦᐆᒡ ᐧᐁᔅ ᒌ ᒥᔅᑕ ᑕᐦᑳᔮᔫ ᑲᔦ ᒌ ᔫᑎᓂᔫ, ᐊᓂᑌ ᒫᒃ ᐧᐄᓂᐯᑯᐦᒡ ᒌᔑ ᐱᒥᐱᒎᒡ ᓀᑌ ᐃᔑ ᑕᐦᑯᐦᑖᒍᐧᐃᓐ ᒋᓴᓲᐲᔫ ᐊᓂᑌ ᑳ ᐃᐦᑖᑯᓂᔨᐧᑳᐤ ᐱᔨᓐ ᐸᒋᔥᑕᐦᐧᐋᑲᓐᐦ᙮ ᓇᐸᒋᑖᐹᓈᔅᑯᐦᒡ ᒌ ᑌᐦᑕᐴ ᐧᕌᔅ ᐁ ᐅᑖᐹᑎᑯᐨ ᐊᑎᒻ᙮ ᐊᓂᑕ ᒫᒃ ᐧᐋᔅᑲ ᐁ ᐃᐦᑖᐨ ᓈᔅᒡ ᐁ ᐧᐋᔅᑲᒫᑯᓂᑳᒡ ᐊᓂᑌ ᐁ ᐊᐃᔅᐹᑲᒋᐦᑎᐦᒡ, ᐁᒄ ᐊᓂᔫ ᐅᑌᒧᐧᐋᐤ, ᐄᔅᒌᒣᐅᑎᒻᐦ ᒌ ᐋᔮᐧᐁᐅᒡ ᓈᔅᒡ ᓲᐦᒃ ᐁ ᐱᒥᐸᐦᑖᔨᐧᑖᐤ ᑰᓐᐦ ᐁ ᐸᐦᒋᔑᓂᔨᒡ ᐊᓂᑌ ᐁᒥᓃ ᐁ ᐃᐦᑖᐨ, ᐅᒧᔔᒻ ᐧᐄ ᒌ ᐱᒥᐸᐦᑖᔫ ᐅᐦᐱᒣ ᐊᓂᑕ ᐊᓂᔫᐦ ᓇᐸᒋᑖᐹᓈᔅᑯ᙮ ᐋᔅᑰ ᒌ ᑌᐦᒋᐹᔨᐦᐆ ᐊᓂᑕ ᐅᑖᐹᓈᔅᑯᐦᒡ ᒎᔑᐦᑖᒡ ᐁ ᐊᔦᔅᑯᓲᐨ ᒥᒄ ᑮᐹ ᐧᐁᐃᐱᔅᒌᔥ᙮

ᐁᒄ ᒫᒃ ᐁ ᐃᑎᑯᐨ, “ᑲᓇᐧᐋᐸᒥᒡ ᒫ,” ᐃᐧᑌᐤ ᐊᓂᔫ ᑳᐦᑌᐦᒋᐸᔨᐦᐅᐨ ᐅᑖᐹᓈᔅᑯᐦᒡ, “ᓄᐧᐊᒡ ᐄᐧᐹᐦᑳᐅᒡ᙮ ᒋᔅᒉᔨᐦᑕᒧᒡ ᑖᓂᑕ ᐁ ᐸᐸᑲᑕᓂᔨᒡ ᐁᒄ ᓇᒧᐃ ᒋᑲ ᐅᐦᒋ ᐃᔅᐸᐦᑖᐅᒡ ᐊᓂᑌ᙮ ᒋᑲᒌ ᐃᔑᑖᐹᑎᑯᓅᒡ ᐊᓂᑌ ᐁ ᐃᐦᑖᔨᐧᑖᐤᐦ ᓂᑕᐦᐄᐲᐦ ᒋᓱᔮᒎᓐ ᐊᓂᑕ ᑲᔦ ᑯᔥᑖᑎᑯᓐ ᒥᒄ ᒫᒃ ᒋᑲᒌ ᐃᐦᑑᒡ ᐧᐁᔑᓐ᙮”

ᓇᒧᐃ ᐅᐦᒋ ᐧᐄ ᐊᔦᔅᑯᐦᐁᐤ ᐊᓂᔫᐦ ᐊᑎᒻᐦ ᐁᒄ ᐧᐄᐸᒡ ᑳ ᐋᒥᐱᐦᑖᐨ ᐊᓂᑕ ᐅᑖᐹᓈᔅᑯᐦᒡ ᐁᒄ ᒦᓐ ᑳ ᒋᐦᒋᐸᒑᔑᐨ ᐊᓂᑕ ᐅᐦᐱᒣ᙮

ᐃᔅᑯᑕᒃ ᒫᒃ ᐧᐁᑎᐦᑖᐧᑖᐤ ᐯᔭᒄ ᐊᓂᔫᐦ ᐊᐦᐄᐲᐦ ᐁᒄ ᑳ ᐋᒦᐨ ᐧᕌᔅ ᐊᓂᑕ

Quand Rose était petite, qu'elle n'allait pas encore à l'école, son grand-père et elle s'emmitouflaient pour se protéger du vent froid de la baie et prenaient le traîneau à chiens pour traverser la baie d'Hudson et remonter La Grande Rivière afin de vérifier les filets de pêche. Rose se perchait sur le traîneau, le soleil scintillait sur les congères autour d'elle, les huskies frénétiques faisaient voler la neige devant elle et son grand-père courait le long du traîneau. Parfois, il sautait sur le traîneau pour prendre une minute ou deux de repos.

When Rose was a young girl, not yet in school, she and her grandfather swaddled against the cold bay wind and took the dogsled over Hudson Bay and up the La Grande River to check the fishnets. Rose perched up on the sled, the sun glinted off snowdrifts around her, the frenzied huskies kicked up snow in front of her, and her grandfather ran alongside the sled. Sometimes he jumped on for a minute or two of rest.

« Regarde, disait-il alors, tu peux voir à quel point les chiens sont intelligents. Ils savent où la glace est mince et ils l'évitent. Nous pouvons aller jusqu'à mes filets de rivière, où l'eau coule plus vite et où la glace est plus dangereuse, seulement grâce à eux ».

"Look," he said then, "you can see how smart the dogs are. They know where the ice is thin and they avoid it. We can go to my river nets, where the water runs faster and the ice is more dangerous, only because of them."

Cependant, il ne voulait pas fatiguer les huskies avec son poids supplémentaire, et il sautait bientôt du traîneau pour courir à grandes enjambées à ses côtés.

He didn't want to tire the huskies with his extra weight, though, and soon hopped off the sled again to lope along beside.

Lorsqu'ils atteignaient un filet de pêche, Rose descendait du traîneau et les chiens

When they reached a fishnet, Rose climbed down from the sled and the dogs

ᐊᓂᒌ ᐊᑎᒧᒡ, ᐋᑯᐦ ᑳ ᒌ ᓈᑎᐦᐄᐹᔨᒡᐦ ᐊᓂᔮᐦ ᐅᒧᔓᒻᐦ ᐋᑦ ᓈᐅᔥ ᒌᐦ ᐱᒥᐱᐦᑖᔨᒡᐦ᙮ ᓈᔥᒡ ᐋᐦ ᒌᐦ ᑯᓯᐧᑳᐹᐧᐋᔨᒡᐦ ᐊᓂᔮᐦ ᐃᐦᐄᐲᐦ ᐋᐦ ᒥᔅᑯᒦᐧᐃᔨᒡᐦ ᑮᔮᐦ ᐋᐦ ᓂᐲᐧᐃᔨᒡᐦ ᑮᔮᐦ ᐋᐦ ᒋᑭᒧᔨᒡᐦ ᐅᐱᑎᐦᐧᐃᔮᑭᓂᐧᐋᐤᐦ ᒥᒄ ᑳ ᒌ ᐧᐋᒋᔨᑯᔨᒡᐦ ᐅᒧᔓᒻᐦ ᑮᔮᐦ ᑳ ᒌ ᒥᒫᔥᑭᐧᐃᔨᑯᔨᒡᐦ ᐊᓂᔮᐦ ᐃᐦᐄᐲᐦ᙮᙮ ᑲ ᒌ ᒥᓂᓈᔨᒡᐦ ᐊᓂᔮᐦ ᓂᒫᔅᐦ ᑮᔮᐦ ᑳ ᒌᐦ ᐅᑖᒥᔥᑎᑳᓈᔓᒫᔨᐦᒡ ᐋᔥᒄ ᐋᔨᐧᐃᑳᓂᐦᐄ ᐊᓂᑎᐦ ᒥᔅᑯᒦᐦᒡ, ᑳ ᒌ ᐧᐋᐧᐋᒋᐱᔨᐦᐋᔨᒡᐦ ᑮᔮᐦ ᑳ ᒌ ᐴᓯᐦᐋᔨᒡᐦ ᐊᓂᑖᐦ ᐲᐦᒡ ᐅᑖᐹᓈᔅᑯᐦᒡ᙮ ᒦᓐ ᑳ ᒌ ᐴᓯᑦ ᒍᔅ ᐅᑖᐹᓈᔅᑯᐦᒡ ᐋᑯᐦ ᒦᓐ ᑳ ᒌ ᒋᐦᒋᐱᔨᒡ, ᒦᓐ ᑯᑎᒃᐦ ᐃᐦᐄᐲᐦ ᒑ ᓈᑎᐦᐧᐋᒡ, ᐅᐦᐱᒫ ᐋᐦ ᐱᒥᐱᐦᑖᔨᒡᐦ ᐅᒧᔓᒻᐦ᙮

ᑳᐦ ᒌᐧᐋᐱᔨᐧᑖᐤᐦ ᐋᑎ ᐅᑖᑯᓱᔨᒡᐦ, ᑳ ᒌ ᐊᑎᒧᑖᓂᐧᐋᔨᒡᐦ ᐅᒧᔓᒻᐦ ᐅᔅᑭᓐᐦ, ᐧᐄᔮᓯᔨᐤ ᑮᔮᐦ ᐅᔥᐧᑳᔥᐦ ᒑ ᒦᒋᓯᔨᐦ ᐊᑎᒻᐦ᙮

“ᐄᓱᓈᑯᓐ ᐧᐋᔥ ᒨᔥ ᑯᐃᔅᒄ ᒑ ᐊᓱᒫᑭᓂᐅᐧᐃᒡ ᐊᑎᒧᒡ,” ᐄᑎᑰ ᒍᔅ ᐅᒻᔓᒻᐦ, “ᐧᐋᓱᑯᒥᒌᓱᑳᐤᐦ, ᓃᐧᔖᐤ ᐹᔨᑯᒌᓱᑳᐤᐦ, ᑮᔮᐦ ᓂᒥᔮᔨᐤ ᒥᒄ ᐊᓂᔮ ᑳᓱᑳᔨᒡ ᐃᔮᐱᒥᐦᐋᑭᓂᐅᐧᐃᒡ᙮ ᐊᐧᑳᐧᐄ ᓂᐦᑖ ᓂᑎᐧᐄ ᐃᐦᑐᑎᐤ ᐊᑎᒻ; ᒥᓯᐧᐋ ᒋᑭ ᒋᔥᑖᔨᒫᐧᐃᒡ ᐊᑎᒧᒡ᙮”

ᐹᑎᔥ ᒥᓯᐧᐋ ᑳ ᐊᓱᒫᑦ ᐊᓂᔮᐦ ᐊᑎᒻᐦ ᐄᔮᒄ ᑳ ᐅᐧᐋᔨᐱᑦ ᑮᔮᐦ ᑳ ᐋᔨᐧᐋᓱᑦ᙮

ᓈᐱᓂᔨᒡᐦ, ᐧᐋᐧᐊᔫᑎᓰᐧᑖᐤᐦ ᓂᒫᓯᒡ, ᑳ ᒌ ᐧᐄᒋᐦᐋᑦ ᒍᔅ ᐅᐦᑯᒻᐦ ᐋᐦ ᐹᐧᓵᔨᒡᐦ ᓂᒫᔅᐦ ᑮᔮᐦ

ᐅᑖᐹᓈᔅᑯᐦᒡ, ᑳ ᐊᔪᐧᐁᓰᐧᑖᐤ ᐊᓂᒌ ᐊᑎᒧᒡ ᐁᒄ ᐅᒧᔔᒻ ᑳ ᓈᑕᐦᐄᐯᔨᒡ ᐁᒌ ᒫᒃ ᒥᔅᑕᒋᐦᒋᐸᐦᑖᔨᒡ᙮ ᓈᔅᒡ ᐁ ᑯᓱᑯᑎᑦ ᐊᓐ ᐊᐦᐊᐲ ᐁ ᐃᔅᐱᔅ ᒥᐦᒉᑎᐧᑖᐤ ᓇᒣᓯᒡ ᑲᔦ ᒫᒃ ᐁ ᑯᓱᐧᑳᐧᐹᐧᐁᑦ ᑲᔦ ᐁ ᒥᔅᑯᒦᐅᑦ ᐊᓐ ᐊᐦᐊᐲ ᐊᓂᔫ ᒫᒃ ᐁ ᐅᒋᐱᑖᑦ ᓄᐧᐊᒡ ᐧᐋᒋᓱᐤ ᐁ ᔖᐸᔨᐦᐅᑦ ᓄᐧᐊᒡ ᒌ ᐋᐸᑎᓰᒪᑲᓂᔫᐦ ᐅᔅᐱᑐᓐᐦ ᑲᔦ ᐅᔅᑳᑦᐦ᙮ ᑳ ᒉᒋᑯᓈᑦ ᒥᓯᐧᐁ ᐊᓂᔫᐦ ᓇᒣᔅ, ᐊᓂᔫᐦ ᐁᔅᒄ ᐁᒌ ᐄᓃᐧᐃᔨᒡ ᒌ ᐅᑖᒥᓱᒣᐤ ᐊᓂᑌ ᐃᓱ ᒪᔅᑯᒦᐦᒡ ᒉᒌ ᓂᐱᔨᒡ ᐁᒄ ᑳ ᐱᔅᐧᑫᔦᒋᐱᑖᑦ ᐅᑖᐹᓈᔅᑯᐦᒡ ᒥᓯᐧᐁ ᐊᓂᔫᐦ ᓀᒣᔅ᙮ ᐁᒄ ᒦᓐ ᑳ ᑕᐦᑯᐦᑖᐦᑕᐧᐄᑦ ᐧᒑᔅ ᐅᓂᔫᐦ ᐅᑖᐹᓈᔅᒄ ᐁᒄ ᑳ ᒫᒌᐧᑖᐤ ᑯᑕᒃ ᐊᐦᐊᐲᐦ ᑫ ᓂᑐᐧᐋᐦᐋᐧᑖᐤ, ᐁᒄ ᐊᓂᔫᐦ ᐅᒧᔔᒻ ᐅᐦᐱᒣ ᐊᓂᔫᐦ ᐅᑖᐹᓈᔅᒄ ᒌ ᐱᒥᐸᐦᑖᔫᐦ᙮

ᐃᔅᑯᑕᒃ ᑌᑯᓱᐦᐧᑳᐤ ᐅᑕᐧᑲᒋᐦᒎᐅᑲᒥᑯᐧᐊᐦᒡ ᐁᒄ ᑳ ᒥᔅᑕ ᐱᒥᓇᐧᐁᔨᒡ ᐅᒧᔔᒻ ᐅᑌᒻᐦ ᐁ ᐱᒥᓅᑖᑦ, ᐅᔅᑲᓐᐦ ᑲᔦ ᐧᐄᔮᓯᔫ ᒌ ᐅᔕᒻ ᐁᒄ ᑳ ᐧᐋᐸᔫᒥᓈᐦᐴᐦᑲᐦᑕᒃ ᐊᓂᔫ ᐊᔅᒋᐦᑯᔫ᙮

“ᒋᑲ ᒥᔫᐦᑯᐧᐋᐅᒡ ᐧᐁᔥ ᐊᑎᒧᒡ,” ᒌ ᐃᑎᑰ, “ᒣᓯᑯᒻ ᒌᓱᑳᐤ ᒋᑲ ᐊᓴᒫᐅᒡ ᒫᒃ ᓃᐧᔖᐤ ᒋᑲᒌ ᐊᓴᒫᐅᒡ ᓇᒧᐃ ᒥᒄ ᐊᓂᑕ ᒉ ᐅᑖᐯᐧᑖᐤ᙮ ᐁᑳᐧᐄ ᐧᐄᔅᑳᒡ ᒋᑲ ᐅᐦᒋ ᐋᐦᑯᐦᐋᐅᒡ; ᒥᓯᐧᐁ ᐁ ᑕᓯᐧᑖᐤ ᒋᑲᐧᐄ ᒥᔫᐦᒎᑕᐧᐋᐅᒡ᙮”

ᐹᑎᔅ ᒫᒃ ᑳ ᐊᓴᒫᑦ ᐅᑌᒻ ᐁᒄ ᔮᒄ ᑳ ᒦᒋᓯᑦ ᐧᐄᔭ᙮

ᐁ ᓃᐱᓃᒡ, ᐊᓂᑕᐦ ᐧᐃᔦᔫᑎᓯᔨᒡ ᓇᒣᔅ, ᒌ ᐧᐋᐧᐄᒋᐦᐁᐤ ᐧᒑᔅ ᐅᐦᑯᒻ ᐁ ᐅᓱᐦᑖᔨᒡ

se reposaient pendant que son grand-père, après toute cette course, remontait la prise. Le filet était si lourd de la glace, d'eau et de poissons que son corps se penchait sur un angle vers l'arrière et ses bras et ses jambes se tendaient sous le poids de celui-ci. Il démêlait les poissons du filet, les frappaient sur la glace pour les tuer rapidement, les emballait et attachait les paquets au traîneau. Rose remontait sur le dessus de la charge et ils repartaient, vers le filet suivant, son grand-père courant à côté.

rested while her grandfather, after all that running, heaved up the catch. The net was so heavy with ice and water and fish that his body leaned back on an angle and his arms and legs strained with the weight of it. He untangled the fish from the net, bashed them on the ice to kill them quickly, bundled them and lashed the bundle to the sled. Rose climbed back on top of the load, and they were off again, on to the next net, grandfather running beside.

De retour au camp en fin de journée, son grand-père préparait un gros repas avec des os, de la viande et du riz pour les chiens.

Back at the cabin at the end of the day, her grandfather cooked up a big meal with bones and meat and rice for the dogs.

« Tu dois bien nourrir les chiens, disait-il, tous les jours, deux fois par jour, et pas seulement les jours où ils tirent le traîneau. Ne sois jamais cruel envers un chien, tu dois respecter chacun d'eux ».

"You must feed dogs well," he said. "Every day, twice a day, and not only on the days they pull the sled. Never be cruel to a dog; you have to respect each one."

Ce n'était qu'après avoir nourri les chiens que lui-même s'asseyait et se reposait.

Only after the dogs were fed did he sit down himself and rest.

En été, lorsque le poisson était plus abondant, Rose aidait sa grand-mère

In the summers, when fish were more plentiful, Rose helped her grandmother

ᐊᓂᑎᐦ ᒑ ᐊᑯᔮᒡ ᒥᔥᑎᒄᐦ ᐋᐦ ᐋᐱᒋᐦᑖᒡ ᑮᔮᐦ ᐅᑎᐲᐦ ᐋᐦ ᒫᑯᐱᒋᑳᒑᒡ᙮ ᐊᓂᑎᐦ ᐋᓈᐦᒡ ᑳ ᒌ ᑯᑎᐧᐋᒡ ᑮᔮᐦ ᐋᑯᑎᐦ ᑳ ᒌ ᐊᑯᔮᒡ ᐊᓂᔮᐦ ᓂᒫᔥᑖᒄᐦ ᒑ ᑳᐦᒋᓯᔮᒡᐦ ᑮᔮᐦ ᒑ ᑎᑭᓯᔮᒡᐦ ᐊᓂᑎᐦ ᐋᐦ ᐋᐧᑳᐱᐦᑖᔮᒡ᙮ ᐧᐄᐦᑳᔮᐦᒡ ᑳ ᒌ ᐲᐦᑎᐦᐧᐋᑦ ᑮᔮᐦ ᐋᑯᐦ ᐊᓂᑖᐦ ᑳᐱᔅᒋᑯᐹᔮᒡ ᐋᑯᑎᐦ ᑳ ᒌᐦ ᐲᐦᑎᐦᐧᐋᒡ᙮ ᐋᑯᐦ ᐊᓂᑖᐦ ᒑ ᐊᔥᑎᐦᒋᑯᔮᒡᐦ ᐊᓂᔮᐦ ᐅᐦᑯᒻᐦ ᐊᓂᑖᐦ ᐄᑖᒥᐦᒡ ᐊᔅᒌᐦᒡ ᐋᑯᑖᐦ ᑳ ᒌ ᐄᑐᐦᑎᐦᐋᒡ ᐊᓂᑖᐦ ᐋᐦ ᒌᐦ ᐃᔮᐅᐦᑭᐦᐄᒑᔮᒡᐦ ᑮᔮᐦ ᐊᔅᒌᔮᐤ ᐋᐦ ᒌᐦ ᐊᔅᑖᔮᒡᐦ ᒑ ᑎᐦᑳᔑᔮᒡ ᐊᓂᑎᐦ ᐋᐦ ᐄᐦᑎᔮᒡ ᐊᓂᔮᐦ ᓂᒫᔥᑖᒄᐦ ᑮᔮᐦ ᐊᓯᓃᐦ ᑳ ᒌ ᐊᔥᑖᒡ ᐊᓂᑎᐦ ᑎᐦᑯᐦᒡ ᐋᐦ ᑯᓯᑯᓂᔮᒡᐦ ᐋᑳ ᒑ ᒌᐦ ᐱᒫᔮᐦᑎᒥᔮᒡᐦ ᐊᑎᒻᐦ ᑮᔮᐦ ᒥᐦᐄᐦᑭᓐᐦ᙮

ᒋᐎᓂᑐᐦᐅᐧᐃᓂᔮᐤ ᑮᔮᐦ ᐊᓂᔮ ᐋᐦ ᐃᔮᐱᐎᔑᔮᒡ ᓂᑐᐦᐅᐧᐃᓂᔮᐤ = ᒨᔅᐦ, ᑮᔮᐦ ᐊᑎᒄᐦ ᑮᔮᐦ ᐱᔮᐤᐦ ᑮᔮᐦ ᐧᐋᐳᔥᐦ = ᒥᒄ ᒌᐦ ᐱᒧᐦᑖᔮᐤᐦ ᐅᐦᑯᒻᐦ ᑮᔮᐦ ᐅᒧᐎᒻᐦ ᐋᐦ ᐧᐄᐦ ᓂᐱᐦᐋᔮᒡᐦ, ᑮᔮᐦ ᒫᒃ ᑳ ᒌ ᑖᐱᐧᑳᔮᒡᐦ ᑮᔮᐦ ᒫᒃ ᑲ ᒌ ᐧᐃᓂᐦᐋᒧᐧᐋᔮᒡᐦ ᑮᔮᐦ ᐋᔑᑯᒥᑎᐧᐃᔥᑖᐤ ᑳ ᒌ ᓈᑎᐧᑳᔮᒡᐦ ᑮᔮᐦ ᑳ ᒌ ᓈᒋᐧᐃᓂᐦᐄᒑᔮᒡᐦ᙮ ᐊᓂᑖᐦ ᒫᒃ ᐋᑎ ᐄᔥᐧᑳᐱᐦᑖᒌᔑᑳᔮᒡᐦ ᐋᑯᑎᐦ ᑳ ᒌ ᐲᐎᐧᐋᔮᒡᐦ ᐹᔅ ᐅᐦᑯᒻᐦ ᑮᔮᐦ ᔫᒋᓂᔥᐦ ᑳ ᒌ ᐅᔑᐦᐋᔮᒡᐦ᙮ ᐊᓂᑖᐦ ᐊᑖᐧᐋᐅᑭᒥᑯᐦᒡ ᐋᑯᑖᐦ ᑳ ᐅᐦᒋᐱᔮᔮᒡᐦ ᐱᐦᐧᑳᔑᑭᓐᐦ ᑮᔮᐦ ᓂᔮᓂᔫᓐᐦ

ᐸᑯᑕᐧᑳᐧᐋᓂᔫ ᐊᓂᑌ ᑫ ᐹᐧᓵᐧᑖᐤ ᐅᓇᒣᓯᒧᐧᐋᐤᐦ, ᒥᔅᑎᒄ ᐁ ᐋᔮᐱᐐᔥᑯᓯᔮᒡ ᐁ ᐋᐸᒋᐦᐋᐧᑖᐤ ᑲᔦ ᐲᐐᑲᓈᐱᔫ᙮ ᑳ ᐅᔑᐦᑖᐧᑖᐤ ᐁᒄ ᑳ ᑯᑕᐧᐁᐦᑲᐦᑕᐦᐧᑳᐤ ᒋᑲᔥᑳᐦᑎᒄ ᐁ ᐋᐸᒋᐦᑖᐧᑖᐤ ᐁᒄ ᒫᒃ ᑳ ᐊᑯᑖᐧᑖᐤ ᐊᓂᔫᐦ ᐅᓇᒣᓯᒧᐧᐋᐤᐦ ᑫ ᐧᑳᐱᓯᔮᐧᑖᐤᐦ᙮ ᐃᔅᑯᑕᒃ ᑳ ᒌᔑᐧᑳᐱᓯᔮᒡ ᐁᒄ ᑳ ᓈᓃᐦᑎᓈᐧᑖᐤ ᑳ ᐱᔅᐧᑫᔦᒋᓈᐧᑖᐤ ᐸᐦᐧᑫᔑᑲᓐ ᐧᐄᐦᐧᑫᔮᐦᒡ ᐁᒄ ᐱᒥᒋᐧᐊᑎᐦᒡ ᑳ ᐹᐲᐦᑕᐦᐧᑖᐤ᙮ ᒌ ᐃᐦᑕᑯᓂᔫ ᑖᓂᑌ ᑲᒌ ᒋᔅᑲᔥᑖᔮᒡ ᐅᐦᑯᒻᐦ ᒦᒋᒥᔫ ᓂᑖᒥᐦᒡ ᐊᔅᒌᐦᒡ ᐁᑯᑌ ᐊᓂᑌ ᑳ ᓂᑑ ᒋᔅᑲᐦᐋᐧᑖᐤ ᐊᓂᔫᐦ ᓇᒣᔅ᙮ ᓂᔮᓂᐐᑉ ᒥᓂᑯᔥ ᒌ ᐃᔅᐱᔑᓈᑯᓂᔫ ᐊᓂᑌ ᑳ ᐃᑐᐦᑕᐦᐧᑖᐤ᙮ ᐊᓂᑕ ᒫᒃ ᐊᓂᔫ ᑳ ᒨᓇᐦᐊᒥᔮᒡ ᐅᐦᑯᒻ ᐊᔅᒋᔫ ᒌ ᐋᔥᑖᔫ ᓄᑌ ᓂᑖᒥᐦᒡᒻ ᐁᐅᒄ ᑮᐸ ᐊᓐ ᒌᐎᓂᑲᓐ᙮ ᑳ ᐊᐦᐋᐧᑖᐤ ᐊᓂᔫᐦ ᐅᓇᒣᓯᒧᐧᐋᐤᐦ ᐊᓂᑕ ᐊᓂᔫ ᑳ ᐸᑯᓄᔮᒡ ᐊᔅᒌᒡ ᐊᓂᑕ ᐁ ᑕᐦᑳᔮᒡ ᐁᒄ ᐊᓯᓃᐦ ᑳ ᐋᐸᒋᐦᐋᐧᑖᐤ ᐁ ᐊᑯᓇᐦᐧᐋᐧᑖᐤ ᐊᓂᔫ ᓇᒣᔅ ᐁᑳ ᑫᒌ ᐱᑫᔮᒫᔮᒡ ᒫᐦᐄᐦᑲᓐᐦ᙮

ᐊᐧᐁᔩᓯᒡ ᑳ ᐊᐱᔒᔑᐧᑖᐤ ᑲᔦ ᑳ ᒥᓯᒋᔥᑎᐧᑖᐤ = ᒨᔅ, ᐊᑎᐦᒄ, ᐱᔦᐤ ᑲᔦ ᐧᐋᐳᔥ = ᒌ ᐱᒧᐦᑌᐅᒡ ᐁ ᓈᓂᑐᐧᐁᔮᒫᐧᑖᐤ, ᒌ ᐊᑯᑖᐅᒡ ᑲᔦ ᒌ ᐧᐊᓇᐦᐄᑫᐅᒡ ᒣᓯᑯᒻ ᑑᔥᑌᐤ ᒫᒃ ᒌ ᓈᑕᐧᑫᐅᒡ ᑲᔦ ᒌ ᓈᒋᐧᐊᓂᐦᐄᑫᐅᒡ᙮ ᒌ ᐱᒥᓄᐧᐁᔫ ᐧᓵᔅ ᐅᐦᑯᒻ ᐧᐃᔮᓯᔫ ᐁ ᑕᑲᔅᒥᔮᒡ ᑲᔦ ᔩᐹᐃᐦ ᓃᔮᓂᑯᑌᒡ ᒌ ᐅᔑᐦᐁᐤ ᑫᐧᑳᔫ ᐁ ᐱᒥᓄᐧᐁᑦ᙮ ᐊᑖᐧᐋᐅᑲᒥᑯᐦᒡ ᒌ ᐅᐦᑎᓄᐅᒡ ᐸᐦᐧᑫᔑᑲᓐᐦ ᐊᓂᑌ ᐅᑌᓈᐦᒡ ᐁᒄ ᐋᔥᑰ, ᐁ ᐃᔅᑯᐸᔮᐦᒡ ᐸᐦᐧᑫᔑᑲᓐᐦ, ᐋᐦᐃᑯᓈᐤᐦ ᒌ ᐅᔑᐦᐁᐤ ᐁᒄ ᐅᒦᒋᒥᐦᒡ ᑲᒌ ᐊᑯᐦᒋᒫᑦ ᐊᐧᐁᓐ ᐁ ᒦᒋᓱᑦ᙮

à construire un séchoir avec de jeunes arbres et de la babiche. Elles l'étendaient au-dessus d'un feu de bois de vert et, ensemble, elles accrochaient les poissons sur le séchoir pour les fumer jusqu'à ce qu'ils soient bien conservés. Elles enveloppaient le poisson dans un tissu provenant d'un sac de farine et chargeaient les paquets dans des sacs. Puis elles transportaient les sacs sur leur dos jusqu'à la cache de sa grand-mère, un lieu d'entreposage à 15 minutes de là, qu'elle avait creusé en caveau et tapissé de mousse pour l'isolation. Elles plaçaient les paquets de poissons à l'intérieur de la mousse où ils resteraient au frais et empilaient sur les roches les plus lourdes qu'elles pouvaient trouver pour que les loups ne puissent pas les atteindre.

Le gros et le petit gibier – orignal et caribou, perdrix et lapin – étaient tous chassés à pied ou pris dans des collets et des pièges que ses grands-parents relevaient chaque semaine. Pendant de longs après-midis, la grand-mère de Rose cuisait le gibier en ragoûts à petit feu et faisait flotter des boulettes de pâte dans les sauces brunes. La farine avait été achetée en ville et parfois, quand il y en avait assez, elle faisait de la bannique pour saucer les jus de cuisson.

build a drying rack from saplings and sinew. They straddled it across a damp-wood fire and together they draped fish over the rack to smoke until they were well-preserved. They wrapped the fish up in a cloth from a flour sack and loaded the bundles into sacks. Then they carted the sacks on their backs to her grandmother's cache, a storage area 15 minutes away that she had dug out underground and lined with moss for insulation. They placed the fish bundles inside the moss where they would stay cool and piled on top the heaviest rocks they could find so the wolves couldn't get at them.

The big and small game – moose and caribou and grouse and rabbit – was all hunted on foot, or caught in snares and traps that her grandparents would walk to every week. Over long afternoons, Rose's grandmother would slow-cook the game into stews and float soft dumplings in the dark gravies. The flour had been purchased in town and sometimes, when there was enough of it, she made bannock to sop up the juices.

ᐋᔅᐱᔭᔭᒡᐦ ᐱᐦᐧᑳᔑᑭᓐᐦ ᐋᐃᐦᑯᓈᐤᐦ ᑳ ᒌ ᐅᔑᐦᐋᔭᒡᐦ ᑖ ᒌᐦ ᐊᑯᐦᒋᒧᒡ ᐊᓂᑎᐦ ᒨᔥᑭᒦᐦᒡ᙮

ᐆᐦᐱᐦᐆᐲᓯᒻ ᐋᑯᒋᒃᐦ ᐋᑯᑎᐦ ᑳ ᒌᐦ ᒧᐧᐃᓯᓈᓂᐧᐃᒡ, ᐋᑯᑎᐦ ᑳ ᒌ ᒥᐧᔩᒡᐦ ᐄᔭᒥᓐᐦ᙮ ᑳ ᑖ ᒋᔅᑐᐦᒑᒡ ᒉᔅ ᐅᐦᑯᒻᐦ ᑭᔩᐦ ᐅᒧᓚᒻᐦ ᐊᔥᑭᓂᒌᔑᑳᐤᐦ ᑳ ᒌ ᒧᐧᐃᓯᒡ᙮ ᑳ ᒌ ᐅᔑᐦᑖᔭᒡᐦ ᐹᔅᒋᐧᐃᔅᐧᐋᓂᔭᐤ ᒉᔅ ᐅᐦᑯᒻᐦ ᐋᔪᐧᐃᒄ ᑳ ᒌ ᔑᐧᓛᐦᐋᒫᒡ, ᑭᔩᐦ ᑳ ᒌ ᐹᓯᒥᔭᒡᐦ ᐱᔥᒡ ᐧᐄᐦᐧᑳᔩᐦᒡ ᐋᐦ ᐲᐦᑎᐦᐋᒥᔭᒡᐦ ᐋᑳ ᑖ ᒌᐦ ᐊᐧᑳᑯᐦᑎᓂᔭᒡᐦ᙮ ᐋᔪᐧᐃᒄ ᐋᑯᐦ ᐊᓂᔩ ᑖ ᐱᐳᓂᔭᒡ ᑖ ᐅᐦᒋ ᒦᒋᒡ ᐊᓂᔩᐦ ᓂᒫᔅᐦ ᑭᔩᐦ ᒦᓂᔥᐦ ᑭᔩᐦ ᐊᓂᔩ ᐧᐄᔩᓯᔭᐤ᙮ ᓂᔩᓂᑯᑑᓐᐦ ᒫᒃ ᑖᐹ ᐅᐦᒋ ᐧᐋᔪᑎᓂᔭᐤ ᒦᒋᒥᔭᐤ ᐋᑯᑎᐦ ᑳ ᒌ ᑭᐧᐃᐦᑭᑖᒡ ᐊᐧᐋᓂᒌ᙮ ᐋᑦ ᑭᔭᐧᐹ ᒌᐦ ᓅᑎᒫᓰᒡ, ᓂᑐᐦᐅᒡ ᑭᔩᐦ ᒧᐧᐃᓯᒡ ᐋᔩᐱᒡ ᓂᒥ ᐅᐦᒋ ᐃᐦᑎᑯᓂᔭᐤ ᓂᔩᓂᑯᑑᓐᐦ ᑖᐧᑳᔭᐤ ᑖ ᒦᒋᓈᓂᐧᐃᐧᐃᔭᒡ ᑭᔩᐦ ᐋᔩᐱᒡ ᒌᐦ ᓅᐦᑖᐱᔪᐧᐃᒡ᙮ ᓈᑖᐦ ᐄᔑ ᐧᐄᓂᐹᑯᐦᒡ ᐋᑯᑖᐦ ᑳ ᒌ ᐄᔅᐱᔭᔭᒡᐦ ᒉᔅ ᐅᒧᓚᒻᐦ ᐋᐦ ᒥᔭᔭᐱᔭᒡᐦ ᑭᔩᐦ ᓂᔩᓂᑯᑑᓐᐦ ᒥᒄ ᐧᐋᐦᑯᓂᒡ ᐊᓂᑖᐦ ᐊᓯᓃᐦᒡ ᑳ ᓂᐦᑖᐅᒋᒡ ᐋᐅᑯᓂᒡ ᑳ ᒌ ᒧᐧᐋᑭᓂᐅᐧᐃᒡ᙮ ᒥᒄ ᑭᔭᐧᐹ ᐋᔥᐱᔥ ᒌᐦ ᐃᐦᑐᑎᐦᒡᐦ ᑖ ᒌᐦ ᐱᒫᒋᐦᐅᒡ ᐋᑯᑖᐦ ᒨᔥ ᑳ ᐃᐦᑎᐦᒡ ᐄᔭᔭᐅᒡ, ᒦᓐ ᒫᒃ ᑳ ᒌ ᐃᐦᑎᑯᐦᒡ ᓂᑐᐦᐅᐧᐃᓐ ᑭᔩᐦ ᓂᒫᔅ ᑭᔩᐦ ᐊᓐ ᒥᓯᐧᐋ ᑖᐧᑳᓐ ᓈᐦᑖᐅᒋᐦᒡ ᐊᓂᑎᐦ ᑖ ᒌᐦ ᐅᐦᒋ ᐱᒫᒋᐦᐅᒡ ᐄᔭᔭᐅᒡ᙮

ᒨᔥ ᒌᐦ ᒥᔫᔩᔩᐦᒌᓈᓂᐆ ᑭᔩᐦ ᒌᐦ ᐃᔩᔭᒥᓯᓈᓂᐆ, ᐋᔥᒄ ᐊᓂᑖᐦ ᐱᑯᑎᔅᑭᒥᒡ ᐋᐦ ᒌᐦ ᐅᐦᒋ ᐱᒫᒋᐦᐅᓈᓂᐧᐃᒡ᙮ ᒨᔥ ᒌ ᐱᐹᒥᔭᐦᑖᐧᐃᒡ ᐊᐧᐋᓂᒌ, ᐊᓂᑖᐦ ᑭᔭᐧᐹ ᐋᑎ

ᐁ ᒌᔥᐧᑳᐱᐦᑖᒌᔑᑳᔭᒡ ᐁᑯᑦ ᑳᒌ ᒫᒌᐧᑖᐤ ᒉ ᓂᑑ ᒫᐅᓯᐧᑖᐤ, ᐁᒥᑖ ᐁ ᐧᐄᒉᐧᐋᑦ ᐅᐦᑯᒻ ᑲᔦ ᐅᐦᑯᒻ᙮ ᐹᑎᔥ ᐁᑳ ᒥᔅᑲᐦᐧᑳᐤ ᐁᒄ ᔩᒄ ᑳᒌ ᒌᐧᐁᐧᑖᐤ᙮ ᐹᔅᒎᔅᐧᐋᓂᔫ ᒌ ᐅᐦᑯᒻ ᑲᔦ ᒦᓂᔥ ᐋᐃᑯᓈᐤ ᒌ ᐅᔑᐦᐁᔫ ᐁᒄ ᐸᔅᒡ ᒌ ᐹᓯᒻ ᒦᐧᐊᑎᐦᒡ ᑳ ᐲᐦᑕᐦᐊᐦᒃ ᐁᑳ ᑫᒌ ᐊᐧᑳᑯᐸᔭᓂᔭᐧᑳᐤᐦ᙮ ᒌ ᒫᐅᒋᐦᑖᐅᒡ ᒦᒋᒥᔫ ᐃᔅᑲᓐ ᐱᐳᓐ ᑫ ᐃᔅᐸᔭᐧᑖᐤ, ᓇᒉᔅ, ᒦᓂᔅ, ᑲᔦ ᓇᓈᐦᑰ ᐁ ᐃᔑᓈᑯᓂᔭᒡ ᐧᐃᔩᔅ ᒦᒋᒥᔫ᙮

ᒌ ᐃᔑᓈᑯᓐ ᐁᑳ ᒥᑐᓐ ᐃᐦᑕᑯᐦᒡ ᒦᒋᒻ ᐊᓂᑌ ᓅᐦᒋᒦᐦᒡ ᐁ ᐃᐦᑖᓅᐦᒡ᙮ ᒨᔥ ᒌ ᐋᔭᒥᓰ ᐊᐧᐁᓐ ᐁ ᓈᓂᑐᐧᐁᔭᐦᑕᐦᒃ ᑫᐧᑳᔦ ᑫ ᒌᒋᑦ᙮ ᒨᔥ ᒌ ᐋᔩᐦᒌᐅᒡ ᐁ ᐋᐸᒋᐦᐄᓯᐧᑖᐤ᙮ ᓇᒧᐃ ᐧᐄᔅᑳᒡ

La cueillette des baies avait lieu au mois d'août, lorsque les bleuets étaient d'un sombre bleu marin et étaient devenus sucrées au soleil. Rose et ses grands-parents sortaient l'après-midi et cueillaient tout ce qu'ils pouvaient trouver. Sa grand-mère faisait bouillir certaines baies pour en faire des confitures ou les ajoutaient à des gâteaux, et elle le faisait sécher le reste et le conservait dans un sac de coton où elles ne moisiraient pas. Et avec le poisson, les baies et les autres viandes chassées, ils avaient de quoi manger pendant les longs mois d'hiver.

Certaines années, les années de famine, étaient mauvaises. Même avec la pêche, la chasse et la cueillette des baies, il n'y avait pas assez de nourriture. Alors le grand-père de Rose allait sur les îles dans la baie. Il y avait une plante qui poussait là; Elle ressemblait à une mousse noire et de la laitue. On pouvait la faire bouillir, s'il le fallait, et la manger. Cela aidait à traverser les périodes difficiles.

C'était une vie d'athlète, vivre sur le territoire. On était continuellement en mouvement, juste pour pouvoir manger. Toujours en train de faire quelque chose.

Berry-picking time came around August, when the blueberries were a deep navy and had sweetened in the sun. Rose and her grandparents walked out in the afternoons and picked all they could find. Her grandmother boiled some berries into jams or folded them into cakes, and the rest she dried and preserved in a cotton bag where they wouldn't mould. And with the fish and the berries and other hunted meats, they had food in the long winter months.

Some years, the years of starving, were bad. Even with the fishing and the hunting and the berry-picking, there wasn't enough food. Then Rose's grandfather would go out to the islands in the bay. There was a lichen that grew there; it was something like a black moss and something like lettuce. You could boil it, if you had to, and eat it. It would get you through the bad times.

It was an athletic life, living on the land. You were always moving, just to be able to eat. Always doing something. No one in the area had heard of diabetes then.

ᐅᐧᐃᐦᑖᔭᐦᑎᐦᒡ ᒑ ᒌᐦ ᐅᐦᒋ ᓂᐱᐦᑖᒡ ᒦᒋᒥᔭᐤ᙮ ᑖᐹ ᐅᐦᒋ ᐃᔭᔥᑖᐧᐃᐅᐧᐃᒡ᙮ ᓂᒥ ᓂᐦᑖ ᐅᐦᒋ ᐹᐦᑖᑯᓂᔭᐤ ᐊᐧᐋᓐ ᒑ ᒌᐦ ᔔᑳᐅᐱᔭᑦ᙮

ᐋᑯᑖᐦ ᒫᒃ ᑳ ᐄᔑᓈᑯᓂᔭᒡ ᒍᔅ ᐅᐱᒫᑎᓰᐧᐃᓐ ᐋᐦ ᐧᐄᒑᐧᐋᑦ ᐅᒧᔓᒻᐦ ᐊᑎᒻᐦ ᐋᐦ ᐋᐱᒋᐦᐋᒡ ᐋᓐ ᐱᐧᑳᐦᐄᐹᒡ ᑭᔮᐦ ᐋᐦ ᓈᑎᐦᐄᐹᒡ, ᒑᒃ ᑳ ᐅᑎᐦᒋᐱᔭᔭᒡ ᒍᔅ ᒑ ᐲᐦᒋᒑᑦ ᒋᔅᑯᑎᒫᒎᐦᑭᒥᑯᐦᒡ, ᐋᑯᑎᐦ ᒫᒃ ᑳ ᐧᐋᐱᐦᑎᐦᒃ ᒑᐧᑳᔭᐤ ᐋᐦ ᐊᔑᒫᑭᓂᐅᐧᐃᒡ ᐋᑳ ᓂᐦᑖ ᐅᐦᒋ ᒦᒋᑦ ᐊᓂᑖᐦ ᐧᐄᒋᐧᐋᐦᒡ, ᐱᓭᑭᓀ ᒌᐦ ᐄᔑᓂᐦᑳᑖᔭᐤ ᑭᔮᐦ ᐋᔪᐧᐃᒄ ᑳ ᓂᑎᐧᐋᔭᒫᑭᓂᐧᐃᑦ ᒑ ᒦᒋᑦ = ᒥᒄ ᒫᒃ ᓂᒧᐃ ᒦᒋᒥᐦᒡ ᐅᐦᒋ ᐄᔑᓂᒻ ᒍᔅ᙮ ᒌᐦ ᓈᓈᑭᒋᐦᐋᑭᓂᐤ ᔮᔭᑖ ᒑ ᒋᑖᑦ ᐊᓂᔮ ᑳ ᐊᔑᒫᑭᓂᐧᐃᑦ, ᐋᑳ ᒫᒃ ᒋᑖᒑ ᒌᐦ ᒋᔅᒑᔭᑎᒻ ᒑ ᒋᔅᑐᑖᑭᓂᐧᐃᑦ ᑭᔮᐦ ᒫᒃ ᐋᑳ ᒑ ᐊᔑᒫᑭᓂᐧᐃᑦ ᒦᓐ ᒦᒋᓯᓈᓂᐧᐃᔭᒑ ᑭᔮᐦ ᒫᒃ ᒑ ᐅᑎᑖᒧᐦᐧᐋᑭᓂᐧᐃᑦ ᐹᑎᔥ ᐋᑳ ᒌᐦ ᐧᐃᓂᔥᑳᒑ ᐊᓂᑎᐦ ᐅᐦᒋ ᐅᓂᐹᐧᐃᓂᐦᒡ᙮ ᐋᑯᑎᐦ ᑳ ᒌ ᐱᓯᐧᑳᐱᑦ, ᑳ ᒌ ᐧᐄᐦ ᒋᔅᒋᓰᑎᑎᒃᐦ ᐊᓂᔮ ᒑᐧᑳᔭᐤ ᐋᐦ ᒥᐧᔮᔭᐦᑎᐦᒃ ᐋᐦ ᒋᔅᑯᑎᒫᓯᑦ = ᐋᐦ ᐱᔥᑎᐧᑳᔭᐅᔭᒥᓈᓂᐧᐃᐧᐃᔭᒡ ᑭᔮᐦ ᒫᒃ ᐋᐦ ᑎᑭᓯᑭᓂᐧᐃᐧᐃᔭᒡ ᒑᐧᑳᔭᐤ ᑭᔮᐦ ᒫᒃ ᐋᐦ ᐅᔑᐦᑖᑭᓂᐧᐃᐧᐃᔭᒡ ᒑᐧᑳᔭᐤ = ᐋᑯᑎᐦ ᒥᒄ ᐧᐋᐦᒋ ᒌᐦ ᐃᐦᑐᑎᐦᒃ ᒑ ᒌᐦ ᒦᒋᑦ ᐊᓂᔮ ᒑᐧᑳᔭᐤ ᓈᔥᒡ ᐋᑳ ᐅᐦᒋ ᒦᒋᒥᓈᑯᓂᔭᒡ᙮ ᐋᑯᑖᐦ ᑳ ᒌ ᐄᓯᓈᑯᓯᒡ ᓂᔮᓂᑯᒎᓐᐦ ᐱᔥᒡ ᐄᔭᔭᐅᐊᐧᐋᔑᔑᒡ ᐋᐦ ᐋᑭᑖᐱᔭᔭᒡ ᑭᔮᐦ ᐋᐦ ᐹᑯᒨᒡ ᐅᐦᒋ ᐊᓂᔮ ᒑᐧᑳᔭᐤ ᐋᐦ ᓂᑎᐧᐋᔭᒫᑭᓂᐅᐧᐃᒡ ᒑ ᒦᒋᒡ ᐋᑳ ᓂᐦᑖ ᐅᐦᒋ ᐧᐋᐱᐦᑎᐦᒡᐦ ᑭᔮᐦ ᐅᐦᒋ ᑯᒋᔥᑎᐦᒡᐦ᙮ ᐊᑎᑎᐤ ᓈᔥᒡ ᓂᒥ ᐅᐦᒋ ᐧᐄᐦᑭᓂᔭᐤ ᑳ ᐄᔅᐱᑯᓂᔭᒡ ᐧᐋᐦᑯᓐᐦ ᓂᔮᓂᑯᒎᓐᐦ ᑳ ᒌ ᒦᒋᒡ ᐋᔥᒄ ᐋᐦ ᒌᐦ ᐧᐄᒋᒫᑦ ᐅᒧᔓᒻᐦ ᑭᔮᐦ ᐅᐦᑯᒻᐦ

ᐅᐦᒋ ᐯᐦᑖᑯᓐ ᑫᒌ ᓰᐧᐋᑲᒥᐦᐧᑫᑦ ᐊᐧᐁᓐ᙮

ᐊᓂᔫ ᐯᐳᓂᔭᒡ ᑳᒌ ᐧᐄᑫᐧᐋᑦ ᐅᒧᔔᒻ ᐁ ᓈᑕᐦᐄᐯᔭᒡ ᐊᓂᔫ ᒫᒃ ᒦᓐ ᐯᐳᓂᔭᒡ ᐊᓂᑌ ᔔᐧᐊᓂᐦᒡ ᐁ ᐃᐦᑖᑦ ᐁ ᒋᔅᑯᑕᒫᓰᑦ ᐧᓭᔅ ᒌ ᑲᓇᐧᐋᐸᐦᑕᒻ ᐅᒦᒋᒻ ᐧᐃᔮᑲᓂᐦᒡ ᐁ ᐊᔥᑌᔭᒡ᙮ ᐸᐧᓭᑲᓀ ᒌ ᐃᔑᓂᐦᑳᑕᒥᔫ ᐊᓂᔫ ᒋᔅᑯᑕᒫᑫᓰᐦ ᒌ ᓂᑐᐧᐁᔭᒫᑲᓅ ᒫᒃ ᑫ ᒦᒋᑦ = ᒥᒄ ᒫᒃ ᐧᒣᐦᒡ ᐁᑳ ᑫᒌ ᒦᒋᓈᓅᐦᒡ ᑫᐧᑳᓐ ᒌ ᐃᔑᓇᒻ᙮ ᒌ ᓈᓈᑲᒋᐦᐋᑲᓅ ᒫᒃ; ᐁᑳ ᑫ ᒦᒋᐧᑫ ᒋᑲ ᐃᐦᑕᑯᓂᔫ ᑫ ᐃᔑ ᐧᐊᐧᐁᔑᐦᐋᑲᓅᑦ, ᐁᑳ ᑫ ᐅᐦᒋ ᒥᔮᑲᓅᑦ ᒦᒋᒥᔫ ᒫᒃ ᑫ ᐸᓯᔅᑌᐦᐧᐋᑲᓅᑦ ᐹᑎᔅ ᐁᑳ ᒣᒋᒻ ᒌ ᐧᐊᓂᔅᑳᓂᓯᑌ ᐅᓂᐯᐧᐃᓂᐦᒡ᙮ ᐁᒄ ᑳ ᒋᐸᐦᐊᐦᒃ ᐅᔅᒌᔑᒄᐦ ᑳᐧᐄ ᓈᓂᑑ ᒋᔅᒋᓯᑦ ᑫᐧᑳᔫᐦ ᐊᓂᔫ ᑳ ᒥᔦᔭᐦᑕᒥᐦᐄᑯᑦ ᐊᓂᔫ ᑳ ᒌᔑᑳᔭᒡ = ᒧᐧᐁᐦᒡ ᐊᓂᑕ ᒣᐧᑳᒡ ᑳ ᒋᔅᑯᑕᒫᓯᑦ ᑳᑯᔅᑫᓰᔭᒧᐧᐃᓂᔫ ᐁᒄ ᒫᒃ ᐁ ᐱᒥᓄᐧᐋᓄᔭᒡ ᑲᔦ ᐁ ᐅᔑᐦᑖᑲᓅᔭᒡ ᑫᐧᑳᔫ = ᑳ ᒋᐦᑲᐦᐊᐦᒃ ᐊᓂᔫ ᐸᐧᓭᑲᓀ ᐁ ᒋᔅᑎᓈᐦᐅᑦ ᐁᑳ ᑫ ᐧᐄᐦᒋᔥᑕᐦᒃ ᐁᒄ ᐋᐃᓵᒡ ᑳ ᐋᐸᐦᐊᐦᒃ ᐅᒎᓐ᙮ ᐃᔅᑯᑕᒃ ᒫᒃ ᑫᐸᐦᐊᐦᒃ ᐅᒎᓐ ᒥᔮᑯᐦᑕᐦᒃ ᒫᒃ ᓈᔅᒡ ᒌ ᐧᐄᓴᒋᔅᐱᑕᒻ ᑲᔦ ᒌ ᒋᒧᔥᑳᔫ ᐊᓂᑌ ᐅᒎᓂᐦᒡ᙮ ᐊᓂᑕ ᒫᒃ ᐊᓂᔫ ᑳ ᒦᒋᓯᐧᑖᐤ ᒥᓯᐧᐁ ᐊᓂᒌ ᑯᑕᑲᒡ ᐄᓅ ᐊᐧᐋᔔᒡ ᒌ ᐋᑲᑌᐸᔫᒡ ᑯᑕᑲᒡ ᒌ ᐹᑯᒨᒡ ᐁᑳ ᐧᐄᐦᒋᔥᑕᐦᐧᑳᐤ ᐊᓂᔫ ᒦᒋᒥᔫ ᐁᑳ ᐧᐄᔥᑳᒡ ᐅᐦᒋ ᒦᒋᐧᑖᐤ᙮ ᑫᔅᑎᓈᔥ ᐁᑎᑑ ᐆ ᓇᒧᐃ ᐅᐦᒋ ᐧᐄᐦᑲᓐ ᐃᔅᐱᔅ ᐊᓐ ᐧᐋᐦᑯᓈᐱᔅ ᐧᐁᔅᑳᒡ ᑳᒌ ᒨᐧᐋᑲᓅᑦ ᒣᐧᑳᒡ ᑳ ᐱᒥᐸᔭᐦᒡ ᐁ ᑰᐦᑲᑖᓅᐦᒡ᙮ ᔮᐸᒡ ᒫᒃ ᒌ ᐊᑯᐦᑕᒻ ᐊᓂᔫ ᐧᓭᔅ ᐁᑳ ᓂᑐᐧᐁᔭᑕᐦᒃ ᑫᒌ ᐅᑕᑖᒧᐦᐧᐋᑲᓅᑦ᙮ ᐁᒄ ᑳ ᐃᑌᔭᐦᑕᐦᒃ, ᒥᓯᒋᔅᑎᔮᐤ ᐋᔮᐅᐧᑳᐧᐁᓂᒡ

Personne dans la région n'avait entendu parler du diabète à l'époque.

L'année suivant les promenades en traîneau à chiens jusqu'aux filets de pêche, Rose était assise dans la salle à manger du pensionnat indien et contemplait quelque chose dans son assiette. Les enseignants l'appelaient « brocoli » et Rose était censée le manger – mais cela ne ressemblait pas à de la nourriture. Cependant, on la surveillait : si elle ne finissait pas son assiette, elle serait punie et soit affamée, soit battue, jusqu'à ce qu'elle ne puisse plus sortir du lit. Alors elle ferma les yeux, essaya de penser aux moments de sa journée scolaire qu'elle aimait – comme le cours de français, le cours de pâtisserie et les travaux manuels – et elle planta sa fourchette dans la vile tige de brocoli et se força à ouvrir la bouche. Lorsqu'elle la referma, des jus amers giclèrent sur sa langue et, en quelques secondes, le brocoli se transforma en une bouillie révoltante. Tout autour d'elle, dans la salle à manger, les enfants cris avaient des haut-le-cœur et vomissaient à cause de cette étrange nourriture. Ce devait être pire que cette plante moussue noire que ses grands-parents avaient mangée à l'époque de la famine. Toutefois, Rose

The year after the dogsled rides to the fishnets, Rose sat in the residential school dining room contemplating something on her plate. The teachers called it "broccoli" and Rose was supposed to eat it – but it didn't look like food. She was being watched, though: if she didn't clean her plate she would be punished and either starved or beaten until she couldn't get out of bed. And so she closed her eyes, tried to think about the parts of her school day that she enjoyed – like French class and baking class and handicrafts – and she stabbed her fork into that vile broccoli stem and willed her mouth to open. When she closed it, bitter juices squirted across her tongue and in seconds the broccoli became a revolting mush. All around her in the dining room, Cree kids were gagging and vomiting at the strange food. This had to be worse than that black lichen her grandparents had eaten in the starving times. But Rose forced it down and avoided a beating. *When I grow up*, she thought, *I will have kids. And I will never force them to eat broccoli*. In those years, there was still no talk of diabetes.

ᐧᐋᐦ ᒦᒋᓯᓈᓂᐧᐃᐧᐃᔨᒡᐦ. ᐋᑯᐦ ᑳ ᒌ ᑯᐦᑎᐦᒃ ᐊᓂᔮ ᑳ ᐊᔑᒫᑭᓂᐧᐃᑦ ᐋᑲ ᓂᑎᐧᐋᔨᐦᑎᐦᒃ ᒑ ᐅᑎᑖᒎᐦᐧᐋᑭᓂᐧᐃᑦ. ᒋᔗᔨᔨᐅᐧᐃᔮᓈ, ᐄᑖᔨᐦᑎᒻ, ᐃᔮᐅᐧᑳᐧᐋ ᒫᒃ ᐊᐧᐋᔑᔑᒡ, ᓂᒧᐃ ᓂᐦᑖ ᓂᑭ ᐊᔑᒫᐧᐃᒡ ᐱᐧᓀᑭᑖ. ᐅᔮ ᒫᒃ ᒫᐧᑳᒡ ᐅᑎᐦ ᑳ ᐃᐦᑖᑦ ᐋᔥᑯ ᓂᒧᐃ ᓂᐦᑖ ᐅᐦᒋ ᐃᔮᔨᐧᒫᐅᐦᐄᐧᐋᐤ ᐋᐦ ᐚᑳᐅᐱᔨᓈᓂᐧᐃᒡ.

ᒫᒃ ᐊᐧᐋᔕᒡ ᓇᒧᐃ ᐧᐄᔅᑳᒡ ᓂᑲ ᐅᐦᒋ ᐋᐃᐦᑲᒥᐦᐋᐅᒡ ᒉᒌ ᒦᒋᐧᑖᐤ ᐸᐧᑫᑲᑖ. ᐊᓂᔦ ᒫᒃ ᐊᓂᑌ ᑳ ᐃᔅᐱᔅ ᐃᐦᑖᑦ ᓇᒧᐃ ᐅᐦᒋ ᒋᔅᑫᔨᐦᑖᑯᓐ ᐁ ᔩᐧᐋᑲᒥᐦᐧᑳᓅᐦᒡ.

ᒐᔅ ᐊᓂᑖᐦ ᒐᐊᓐ=ᐧᓈᑬᓐᑖᐦ ᐋᑯᑖᐦ ᑳ ᒋᔅᑯᑎᒫᓱᑦ ᑳ ᐄᔥᐹᔮᒡ ᒋᔅᑯᑎᒫᑑᑭᒥᑯᐦᒡ, ᒫᐧᑳᒡ ᑯᐧᑖᓱᒥᑎᓂᐤ ᑳ ᐄᒋᔥᑖᔮᒡᐦ ᐋᐦ ᐱᐳᓂᔮᒡᐦ. ᐹᔮᐧᑳᐤ ᐊᓂᑖᐦ ᐋᐦ ᐄᔑ ᐲᐦᒋᒑᑦ ᒦᔫᐅᑭᒥᑯᐦᒡ ᒫᐧᑳᒡ ᒌᐦ ᐃᐦᑖᔮᐤᐦ ᑯᑎᒃᐦ ᐃᔥᐧᑳᔑᔥᐦ: ᒫᐧᑳᒡ ᒌᐦ ᒌᔥᑎᐦᐅᓯᔮᐤᐦ ᐅᐧᐹᒥᔮᒡᐦ ᑳ ᐋᑎ ᐲᐦᒋᒑᑦ. ᑏᐧᐋᐦᒡ ᒌᐦ ᐄᑖᔨᐦᑎᒻ ᒐᔅ ᒥᒋᑐᐦᑯᔮᓂᔮᐤ ᐋᐦ ᐋᐱᒋᐦᑖᔮᒡᐦ, ᐧᐋᐧᐋᒡ ᐅᑎᐦ ᓈᐦᐋᐤ ᐋᐦ ᒋᔅᑯᑎᒫᓱᑦ. ᓂᒥ ᐅᐦᒋ ᒋᒋᔅᑐᑖᐤ ᐊᓂᔮᐦ ᐃᔥᐧᑳᔑᔥᐦ ᑭᔮᐦ ᒥᒄ ᑳ ᒋᔥᑖᐹᐅᑖᑦ ᐅᑎᐦᒌᐦ ᑭᔮᐦ ᑳ ᐋᑎ ᐧᐃᔮᐧᐄᑦ ᒦᓐ ᒑ ᒋᔅᑯᑎᒫᓱᑦ. ᓈᔥᒡ ᒫᒃ ᒦᓐ ᐊᓂᑖᐦ ᐹᑎᒫᐦ ᒫᐧᑳᒡ ᐋᐦ ᒋᔅᑯᑎᒫᓱᑦ ᒐᔅ, ᒑᔅᒋᔫᑎᑎᐧᐋᑦ ᐊᓂᔮᐦ ᐃᔥᐧᑳᔑᔥᐦ ᑳ ᐧᐋᐱᒫᑦ ᐋᐦ ᒌᔥᑎᐦᐅᓯᔮᒡᐦ. ᒫᐧᑳᒡ ᐊᓂᔮ ᐋᐦ ᒋᔅᑯᑎᒫᓱᑦ ᐊᓂᔮᐦ ᐅᒋᔅᑯᑎᒫᒑᔫᒥᐧᐋᐤᐦ ᑳ ᐃᔮᔮᒧᑎᒥᔮᒡᐦ ᐊᓂᑖᐦ ᒌᔮᓈᐦᒡ ᐋᐦ ᐃᔮᔮᐦᑯ ᐲᐦᒋᔮᐤ ᐅᐲᔥᐲᔥᒃ ᑳ ᐄᔑᓂᐦᑳᑖᒡ ᑭᔮᐦ ᐋᔦᐧᐃᑯ ᑳ ᐃᔮᔮᐧᒦᐅᐦᐄᑯᔮᒡᐦ ᑭᔮᐦ ᐋᐦ ᐚᑳᐱᔨᓈᓂᐧᐃᐧᐃᔮᒡ ᑭᔮᐦ ᐋᐦ ᒌᔅᑎᐦᐅᓯᔮᒡᐦ ᐊᐧᐋᔮᐤᐦ ᐄᓐᓯᓇ ᐅᐦᒋ ᐊᓂᔮ ᐋᐦ ᐚᑳᐅᐱᔮᔮᒡᐦ. ᑳᐦ ᒋᔅᒑᔮᐦᑎᐦᒄ ᒐᔅ ᐊᓂᔮᐦ ᑳ ᐧᐋᐱᒫᑦ ᐃᔥᐧᑳᔑᔥᐦ ᐄᓐᓯᓇ ᐋᐦ ᒌᐦ ᒌᔥᑎᐦᐅᓯᔮᒡᐦ ᓂᒦᔮᐤ ᒥᒋᓂᑐᐦᑯᔮᓂᔮᐤ ᑭᔮᐦ ᐋᑲ ᐅᐦᒋ ᐋᐱᒋᐦᑖᔮᒡᐦ ᐊᓂᔮ ᐄᓐᓯᓇ ᐊᑐᒡ

ᐊᓂᔦᐦ ᐊᔅᒌᐤ ᐊᒋᐦᑖᓯᓐ 60 ᑳ ᐃᒋᔥᑌᐧᑳᐤ ᒉᑳᑦ ᒫᒃ ᐁ ᐊᑎ ᒣᐦᒋᐸᔨᐦᐧᑳᐤ, ᐯᔮᐧᑳᐤ ᐁ ᐲᐦᒉᑦ ᐧᓀᔅ ᒦᔫᐅᑲᒥᑯᐦᒡ ᐊᓂᑌ ᐅᒋᔅᑯᑕᒫᒉᐅᑲᒥᑯᐦᒡ ᐊᓂᑌ ᒑᐧᐋᓐ=ᐧᓈᑬᓐᑕ ᑳ ᒋᔅᑯᑕᒫᓱᑦ. ᒌ ᐃᐦᑖᔦ ᐊᓂᑌ ᑯᑕᒃ ᐃᔅᐧᑫᔅ: ᒌ ᐧᐋᐸᒣᐤ ᐁ ᐃᔅᑯᐱᑕᒥᔮᒡ ᐅᑕᑯᐦᐱᔦ, ᑳ ᑌᐦᒋᔥᑖᔮᒡ ᐅᔅᑳᑎᔦ ᐊᓂᑕ ᑳ ᐧᐋᐧᐃᔦᔮᐦᑖᔮᒡ ᐁ ᒥᔅᔮᒡ ᑳᓲᐦᐧᑲᓂᔮᑲᓂᔦ = ᑳ ᐸᒋᔅᑲᐦᐆᓯᔮᒡ ᐅᐧᐹᒦᐦᒡ ᐸᒋᔥᑲᐦᐄᑲᓂᔦ ᐁ ᐋᐸᒋᐦᑖᔮᒡ. ᒪᒋᓂᑐᐦᑯᐦᐄᓰ, ᒌ ᐃᑌᔮᐦᑕᒻ ᐧᓀᔅ, ᐅᑕ ᓂᔮᓂᑕᒻ ᐆ ᒋᔅᑯᑕᒫᒉᐅᑲᒥᑯᐦᒡ ᐁ ᒋᔅᑯᑕᒫᓰᐧᐃᒡ. ᑳ ᑳᔫᐦᑎᐦᒉᑦ ᐧᓀᔅ ᑳ ᐧᐄᐧᐄᑦ ᐊᓂᑕ ᐁᑯ ᒦᓐ ᑳᐤ ᑳ ᓂᑑᐲᐦᒉᑦ ᐊᓂᑌ ᐅᒋᔅᑯᑕᒫᓰᐱᔅᒋᔅᒻ ᐁᑳ ᒉᒋᒻ ᐅᐦᒋ ᐊᔮᒥᐦᐋᑦ ᐊᓂᔦ ᐃᔅᐧᑫᔅ. ᓇᒧᐃ ᒋᓅᔥ ᒌ ᐅᐦᒋ ᒋᔅᒋᔫᑐᑕᐧᐁᐤ ᐊᓂᔦ ᐃᔅᐧᑫᔅ ᒉᐧᑳᒡ ᐁ ᒋᔅᑯᑕᒫᓱᑦ ᑖᓂᑌ ᑳ ᐅᐦᒋ ᓂᐦᑖᐅᒋᓂᔮᒡ ᓇᓈᐦᑯ ᒉᐧᑳᔦ. ᒌ ᐊᔮᒨᒉᔦ ᒥᐲᐲᔅᒃ ᑲᔦ ᒌ ᐋᔮᒨᑕᒻ ᐁ ᔩᐧᐋᑲᒥᐦᐧᑳᓄᔮᒡ ᓅᔥᑕ ᐁ ᐧᐄᒋᐦᐄᑯᑦ ᐁ ᐸᒋᔅᑲᐦᐆᓱᑦ ᐊᐧᐁᓐ ᑳ ᔩᐧᐋᑲᒥᐦᐧᑳᓄᔮᒡ ᑳ ᐋᔮᑦ. ᑳ ᐅᐦᒋ ᒋᔅᒉᔮᐦᑕᐦᒃ ᐧᓀᔅ ᐁᑳ ᐅᐦᒋ ᒪᒋᓂᑐᐦᑯᐦᐄᓯᔮᒡ ᐊᓂᔦ ᑳ ᐸᒋᔅᑲᐦᐆᓯᔮᒡ. ᐁᑳ ᐸᒋᔅᑲᐦᐆᓱᑦ ᒋᐱᒌ ᐃᔑᓈᑯᓂᔦ ᒉᒌ ᓂᐱᑦ. ᐁᐅᒄ ᐅᔦᐦ ᐊᐧᐁᔦᐦ ᒫᐅᒡ ᓅᔥᑕᒻ ᑳ ᒋᔅᒉᔮᒫᑦ ᐧᓀᔅ ᐁ

se força à avaler et évita d'être battue. *Quand je serai grande*, pensa-t-elle, *j'aurai des enfants. Et je ne les forcerai jamais à manger du brocoli.* Dans ces années-là, on ne parlait toujours pas de diabète.

À la fin des années 60, Rose entra dans la salle de bain de son école secondaire à Rouyn-Noranda. Une autre élève était là : une fille qui avait remonté sa jupe, appuyé sa jambe sur la grande fontaine ronde, et qui insérait une aiguille dans la chair de sa cuisse. *Une héroïnomane*, pensa Rose*, ici même, dans mon école secondaire* ! Rose se lava les mains à la fontaine et retourna en classe sans rien dire à la fille. Quelques années plus tard, cependant, en cours de biologie, la jeune fille lui revint à l'esprit. Le professeur parlait du pancréas et d'une maladie appelée diabète qui se traitait par des injections d'insuline. Cette fille s'était injectée non pas de l'héroïne mais de l'insuline, se rendit compte Rose, et sans cela elle serait morte. Elle était la première personne diabétique que Rose ait jamais vue.

In the late '60s, Rose walked into the bathroom of her high school in Rouyn-Noranda. Another student was there: a girl who had hiked up her skirt, propped her leg up on the big round water fountain – and was sliding a needle into the flesh of her thigh. *A heroin addict,* thought Rose, *right here, in my high school!* Rose washed her hands at the fountain and returned to class without saying anything to the girl. A few years later, though, in Biology class, the girl came to mind again. The teacher talked about the pancreas and a disease called diabetes which was treated with injections of insulin. That needle girl had been injecting not heroin but insulin, Rose realized, and without it she would have died. She was the first person with diabetes that Rose ever saw.

ᐧᐄ ᐅᐦᒋ ᒌᐦ ᐱᒫᑎᓯᔭᐤᐦ᙮ ᐋᔪᐧᐃᑯᓐᐦ ᓃᔥᑎᒻ ᑳ ᐧᐋᐱᒫᑦ ᓯᔅ ᐋᐦ ᔖᑳᐅᐱᔭᔭᒡᐦ ᐊᐧᐋᔭᐤᐦ᙮

ᑳᐦ ᐴᓂᒋᔅᑯᑎᒫᓯᑦ ᓯᔅ ᐊᓂᑖᐦ ᐦᐊᑦᓯᓐ ᐯᐃᐦ ᐊᑖᐧᐋᐅᑭᒥᑯᐦᒡ ᒋᓵᓰᐲᐦᒡ ᐋᑯᑖᐦ ᑳᐦ ᐋᐱᑎᓰᑦ᙮ ᒫᐧᑳᒡ ᒫᒃ ᑳ ᐱᒥᐱᔭᒡᐦ ᓃᐧᓵᓯᒥᑎᓂᐤ ᑳ ᐄᒋᔥᑖᒡᐦ ᐋᐦ ᐱᐳᐦᒡᐦ ᓈᔥᑖᐧᐹᐦ ᒥᔥᑏᐦ ᒌᐦ ᐋᐦᒋᐱᔭᐤ ᒑᐧᑳᓐ᙮ ᓂᑐᐦᐅᓰᒡ ᑭᔮᐦ ᓅᑎᒫᔅᓯᐅᒡ ᔅᑮᑑᐦ ᒌᐦ ᐋᐱᒋᐦᐋᐧᐃᒡ ᐋᐦ ᓂᑐᐦᐅᒡ ᑭᔮᐦ ᓂᒥ ᐅᐦᒋ ᐋᐱᒋᐦᐋᐧᐃᒡ ᐊᑎᒻᐦ᙮ ᓈᔥᒡ ᐋᑳ ᐅᐦᒋ ᐃᔮᐱᑖᔭᒫᑭᓂᐅᐧᐃᒡ ᑭᔮᐦ ᓂᒥ ᐅᐦᒋ ᐄᔥᐱᔑ ᒥᔪᓈᓈᑭᒋᐦᐋᑭᓂᐅᐧᐃᒡ ᐊᑎᒧᒡ᙮ ᒨᔭᒻ ᒑᑲᑦ ᒥᓯᐧᐋ ᐊᐧᐋᓐ ᐋᐦ ᐱᒥᐱᔭᑦ ᐊᑖᐧᐋᐅᑭᒥᑯᐦᒡ ᐋᐦ ᐄᑐᐦᑖᑦ, ᐋᑦ ᓈᔥᒡ ᐹᔕᒡ ᐧᐄᐦ ᐄᑐᐦᑖᑦ ᐊᐧᐋᓐ ᐋᔮᐱᒡ ᒌᐦ ᐱᒥᐱᔭᐤ ᑭᔮᐦ ᓈᓈᓂᒌᒻ ᑳ ᐋᑎᒥᐦᒑᑎᒡ ᐅᑖᐹᓈᔅᑯᒡ ᓂᓈᐦᑰ ᐋᐦ ᐄᓯᓈᑯᓯᒡ᙮ ᐊᓂᑖᐦ ᐊᑖᐧᐋᐅᑭᒥᑯᐦᒡ ᒑᒃ ᑳᐦ ᐊᑖᐧᐋᓂᐧᐃᒡᐦ ᑳᑎᑳᔥᑖᐱᔭᒡᐦ᙮ ᐧᐋᔥ ᐧᐄᐱᒡ ᓂᒥ ᐅᐦᒋ ᐃᐦᑎᑯᓐᐦ ᒫᓐᐦ ᐱᔮᐱᔭᐦᐧᑳᐤᐦ᙮ ᒥᒄ ᒌᐦ ᐹᔭᑯᓐ ᐊᓐ ᑳ ᒌ ᓈᓈᑭᒋᐦᑖᑭᓂᐧᐃᒡ ᐋᐅᒄ ᐊᓐ ᓰ ᐲ ᓰ, ᑭᔮᐦ ᒥᒄ ᐹᔭᐧᑳᐤ ᐋᐦ ᒌᓂᐧᑳᓂᐦᑖᑦ ᐹᔭᑯᒌᔑᑳᐤᐦ ᒌᐦ ᓅᑯᓐ = ᐋᔮᐱᒡ ᓈᔥᒡ ᐋᐦ ᒌᐦ ᒨᒋᐦᐄᑯᒡ ᐊᐧᐋᓂᒌ, ᒥᒄ ᑳ ᒌ ᓈᓈᑭᒋᔥᑖᒡ ᓅᑯᓂᔭᒡᐦ᙮ ᐊᓂᒌ ᒫᒃ ᐊᐧᐋᓂᒌ ᐋᑳ ᐃᔮᒡ ᐊᓂᔮᐦ ᑳᑎᑳᔥᑖᐱᔭᔭᒡᐦ ᐊᓂᑖᐦ ᐊᐧᐋᔭᐤᐦ ᐋᐦ ᐃᔮᔭᒡᐦ ᐋᑯᑖᐦ ᑳ ᒌ ᐄᑐᐦᑖᒡ ᐋᐦ ᐧᐄᐦ ᓈᓈᑭᒋᔥᑖᒡ᙮

ᐊᓂᑖᐦ ᒫᒃ ᐋᐦ ᐋᐱᑎᓰᑦ ᓯᔅ ᒌᐦ ᐧᐄᒐᐱᑎᓰᒫᐤ ᐃᔅᐧᑳᐤ ᐊᓂᑖᐦ ᐄᔭᐦᒡ ᐋᐦ ᐅᐦᒌᔭᒡᐦ, ᐧᐄᓵᐧᐋ

ᓰᐧᐋᑲᒥᐦᐧᑫᔭᒡ᙮

ᒌ ᒌᔑᐦᑖᐤ ᐧᓰᔅ ᐁ ᒋᔅᑯᑕᒫᓯᑦ ᐁᒄ ᑳ ᒥᔅᑲᐦᒃ ᐋᐸᑎᓯᐧᐃᓂᔫ ᐊᓂᑌ ᒋᓵᓰᐲ ᐦᐊᑦᓯᓐ ᑲᒻᐸᓃ ᐊᑖᐧᐋᐅᑲᒥᑯᐦᒡ᙮ ᐁᐅᑰ 70 ᑳ ᐃᒋᔥᑌᐧᑳᐤ ᐊᔅᒌᐤ ᐊᒋᐦᑖᓯᓐ ᓅᐧᐊᒡ ᒫᒃ ᒥᔅᑕᐦᐄ ᐋᐦᒌᐅᐦ ᒌ ᐃᑌᔭᐦᑖᑯᓐ᙮ ᓂᑑᐦᐅᓰᒡ ᑲᔦ ᓅᑕᒣᔅᓰᒡ ᑳᐅᔅᒋᑖᑯᓂᒋᐸᐦᑖᔭᒡ ᓰᔅ ᒌ ᐋᐸᒋᐦᐁᐅᒡ ᐁ ᓂᑑᐦᐄᓯᐧᑖᐤ ᓰᔅ ᓇᒧᐃ ᐊᑎᒻᐦ ᐅᐦᒋ ᐋᐸᒋᐦᐁᐅᒡ ᓇᒧᐃ ᓰᔅ ᐅᐦᒋ ᐱᒥᐸᐦᑖᐅᒡ ᐊᓂᑕ ᐅᐦᐱᒣ ᐅᑖᐹᓈᔅᑯᐦᒡ ᐊᑎᒻ ᐁ ᐅᑖᐯᔭᒡ᙮ ᓰᔅ ᓇᒧᐃ ᐅᐦᒋ ᐃᔅᐱᔅ ᐋᐸᑌᔭᐦᑖᑯᓰᒡ ᐊᑎᒧᒡ ᑲᔦ ᓇᒧᐃ ᐅᐦᒋ ᒥᔫᐦᑯᐧᐋᑲᓅᐧᐃᒡ᙮ ᓇᒧᐃ ᑲᔦ ᐅᐦᒋ ᐱᒧᐦᑌᐤ ᐊᐧᐁᓐ ᐊᑖᐧᐋᐅᑲᒥᑯᐦᒡ ᐁᐧᐄ ᐃᑐᐦᑌᑦ ᒌ ᐱᒥᐸᔫᒡ ᐅᑖᐹᓂᔫ ᐋᑦ ᒥᒄ ᐁ ᐊᐱᔖᔑᔭᒡ ᐁ ᓂᑐᐧᐁᔭᐦᑕᐦᐧᑳᐤ ᐧᐁᑖᒡ ᑲᔦ ᒌ ᒥᐦᑫᓐᐦ ᐅᑖᐹᓐᐦ᙮ ᑫᒃ ᒌ ᐊᑖᐧᐋᓅᐦ ᑳᒪᓯᓈᔅᑌᐸᔭᐦᐧᑳᐤ᙮ ᓅᐧᐊᒡ ᐧᐄᐸᒡ ᒌ ᒣᔅᑎᓂᑲᓅᐦ ᑕᐦᐧᑖᐤ ᐱᔮᐸᔭᐦᐧᑳᐤ ᓰᔅ ᒥᒄ ᑳᒌ ᒣᔅᑎᓂᑲᓅᐦᐧᑳᐤ᙮ ᓰᐲᓰ ᐁᐅᒄ ᒥᒄ ᑳᒌ ᓅᑯᐦᒡ ᐅᔅᑲᒡ ᑳ ᐃᐦᑕᑯᐦᐧᑳᐤ ᑳ ᒪᓯᓈᔅᑌᐸᔭᐦᐧᑳᐤ ᒥᒄ ᐯᔭᐧᑳᐤ ᐁ ᒌᓂᐧᑳᓂᐦᑌᑦ ᐧᐋᒡ ᐁᑯᓐ ᑳ ᐃᔥᐱᔥ ᓅᑯᐦᒡ ᑫᐧᑳᓐ = ᐊᓂᑕ ᒫᒃ ᐊᓐ ᑎᐸᐦᐄᑲᓐ ᑫ ᓅᑯᐦᒡ ᒌ ᐴᓂᔫᒡ ᐊᐧᐁᓂᒌ ᑫᐧᑳᔫ ᐁ ᐃᐦᑑᑕᐦᐧᑳᐤ ᐁᒄ ᑳᒌ ᐲᐦᑫᐧᑖᐤ ᐧᐄᒋᐧᐋᐤ ᒫᒃ ᑯᑕᒃ ᐊᐧᐁᔫ ᐧᐄᒋᔫ ᐁᒄ ᐱᑕᒫ ᑳᒌ ᒪᓯᓈᔅᑌᐸᔭᐦᑖᑲᓅᐦᒡ᙮ ᐁᐅᒄ ᑳ ᐃᑕᐱᐧᑖᐤ ᐁ ᒪᓯᓇᔅᑌᐸᔭᐦᑖᐧᑖᐤ᙮

ᒌ ᐃᐦᑖᐤ ᐄᓅ ᐃᔅᐧᑫᐤ ᐋᐱᐦᑑ ᐧᐁᒥᔅᑎᑰᓰᐤ ᐁᒌ ᐃᒋᔅᑲᓂᓯᑦ, ᐧᐃᔦᔅ 50 ᒌ ᑕᐦᑐᐳᓂᓰ, ᒌ

Rose termina ses études et trouva un emploi au magasin de la Baie d'Hudson de Chisasibi. C'était les années 70, une époque de grands changements. Les chasseurs et les pêcheurs utilisaient des motoneiges pour leur travail et ne couraient plus à côté de traîneaux tirés par des chiens. Beaucoup de chiens n'étaient ni respectés ni n'en prenait-on soin. Les gens du coin ne marchaient plus pour se rendre à l'épicerie ; ils conduisaient même pour les plus petites courses et les pick-ups et les voitures encombraient les rues étroites. Pour la première fois, le magasin commença à offrir des téléviseurs. Les gens les achetaient si rapidement que le magasin ne pouvait plus les garder en stock. La CBC était la seule chaîne à cette époque et elle n'était diffusée qu'une heure par jour, mais quand cette heure arrivait, les gens de toute la ville arrêtaient tout ce qu'ils faisaient pour aller dans leur salon ou dans le salon de quelqu'un qui avait un téléviseur. Et ils demeuraient immobiles pendant une heure entière à regarder l'écran et à écouter les nouvelles.

Une femme Métisse d'environ 50 ans travaillait avec Rose au magasin à

Rose finished her schooling and found work at the Chisasibi Hudson's Bay Store. It was the '70s, a time of big changes. Hunters and fishermen used snowmobiles for their work and no longer ran alongside dog-pulled sleds. Many of the dogs were neither respected nor looked after. Locals didn't walk to the grocery store anymore; they drove for even the smallest errand and trucks and cars crowded the narrow streets. For the first time, the store began to stock televisions. People bought them up so quickly the store couldn't keep them stocked. CBC was the only channel in those days, and it was on for just an hour a day – but when that hour came, people all around town stopped whatever they were doing to go to their living room or the living room of someone who had a TV. And they sat immobile for an entire hour looking at the screen and watching the news.

A Métis lady, about 50 years old, worked with Rose at the store in those days, and

ᓂᔮᔪᒥᑎᓂᐤ ᒌᐦ ᐃᐦᑎᐦᑐᐳᐧᓈᓯᔨᐤᐦ, ᒨᔥ ᓈᔥᒡ ᐋᐦ ᒌᐦ ᐧᐄᐦ ᒥᓂᐦᐧᑳᑦ ᐊᓐ ᐃᔅᐧᑳᐤ᙮ ᐧᐋᔨᐱᔥᒌᔥ ᑳᐦ ᐋᐱᑎᓰᒡᐦ ᐊᓂᑖᐦ ᑳ ᒌ ᐄᑐᐦᑖᑦ ᓂᐲᔨᐤ ᐋᐦ ᓂᑎᐧᐋᐱᐦᑎᐦᒃ ᐃᔮᒄ ᒦᓐ ᑳ ᒌ ᐋᐱᑎᓰᑦ᙮ ᓂᒥ ᓰᐦᒃ ᓈᐅᔥ ᒦᓐ ᑳ ᒌ ᐧᐄᐦ ᒥᓂᐦᐧᑳᑦ᙮ ᓈᔥᒡ ᐋᓯᐦᒡ ᐋᐦ ᒌᐦ ᒥᓂᐦᐧᑳᑦ ᒫᓐ ᐊᔥᑭᓂᒌᔑᑳᐤᐦ, ᒧᔮᓪ ᐋᑲ ᒌᐦ ᑖᐱᓯᒧᑦ ᑳ ᒌ ᐃᐦᑎᒃ ᐋᑦ ᓈᔥᒡ ᐋᓯᐦᒡ ᒥᓂᐦᐧᑳᑦ ᓂᐲᔨᐤ᙮ ᐹᔨᒄ ᐊᓂᔮᐦ ᒦᓐ ᐃᔅᐧᑳᐤᐦ ᑳ ᐧᐄᒑᐱᑎᓰᒪᐤ ᑳᐦ ᐧᐋᐱᒫᑦ ᐋᐦ ᐄᐦᑎᔨᐤᐦ ᐅᔮᐦ ᐃᔅᐧᑳᐤᐦ ᑭᔮᐦ ᐋᔫᐧᐃᒄ ᑳ ᐄᔑ ᒥᐦᑖᔨᒫᑦ ᒧᔮᓪ ᓈᔥᒡ ᐋᐦ ᒋᔑᐱᔨᔨᒡ ᐋᑲ ᐊᑎ ᐧᐋᐱᐦᑎᒥᔨᒡᐦ᙮ ᐊᓂᔮ ᒫᒃ ᑳ ᐄᔑ ᐧᐋᐱᒫᑦ ᐋᐦ ᐄᐦᑎᔨᒡᐦ ᑳᐦ ᐄᑖᑦ ᐋᑯᔥ ᓂᑐᐦᑯᔨᓂᑭᒥᑯᐦᒡ ᒑ ᐄᑐᐦᑖᔨᒡᐦ = ᐋᐦ ᐄᑖᑦ ᐋᐦ ᒌᐦ ᐹᑎᐦᒃ ᐋᐦ ᐃᔮᔨᒡᐦ ᐊᐧᐋᔨᐤᐦ ᐋᐦᑯᓯᐧᐃᓂᔨᐤ ᐊᓂᔮ ᐋ ᐄᐦᑎᒡ ᒧᔮᓪ ᐋᑲ ᒌᐦ ᑖᐱᓯᒧᒡ ᑭᔮᐦ ᓈᓈᓂᒌᓪ ᐋᑲ ᐊᑎ ᐧᐋᐱᐦᑎᐦᒡᐦ᙮ ᐧᑳᔖᓐ ᐃᐦᑎᑯᓄᒋᒑ ᓂᑐᐦᑯᔨᓐ ᒑ ᐧᐄᒋᐦᐄᑯᔨᓐ, ᐄᑖᐤ᙮ ᐹᑎᒫᐦ ᒦᓐ ᑳ ᐹᒋ ᒋᔥᑖᐱᑎᓰᑦ ᐊᓐ ᐃᔅᐧᑳᐤ, ᑳᐦ ᒥᔮᑭᓂᐧᐃᑯᐱᓈ ᒌᔥᑎᐦᐄᑭᓂᔨᐤ ᑭᔮᐦ ᒌᔥᑎᐦᐅᐧᐋᐳᔨᐤ᙮ ᐊᓂᑎᐦ ᔖᐳᓂᑭᓂᐦᒡ ᑳᐦ ᐲᐦᑖᔑᑭᐧᐃᐦᑖᑦ ᐊᓂᔮ ᐄᓐᓯᓚᓐ ᑭᔮᐦ ᑳᐦ ᒌᔥᑎᐦᐅᓯᑦ᙮ ᐋᔑᑯᒥᒌᔑᑳᐤᐦ ᒫᒃ ᐅᔮ ᒌᐦ ᐃᐦᑐᑖᓰ᙮ ᑳᐦ ᐃᔭᑦ, ᐋᔑᑯᒥᒌᔑᑳᐤᐦ ᐋᐅᒄ ᐆ ᒑ ᐃᐦᑐᑖᓯᔮᓐ ᒑ ᐄᔥᐱᔑ ᐱᒫᑎᓯᔮᓐ᙮ ᓂᔭᓂᑯᑑᐦᓐ ᒫᒃ ᐊᑎᑎᐤ ᓈᑎᐧᐋᔨᐦᑎᒧᒥᑭᓂᔨᒡᐦ ᐅᔮᐦᒡ ᐊᓂᔮ ᐄᓐᓯᓚᓐ, ᑳ ᒌ ᓈᓈᒥᐱᔨᑦ ᑎᐧᐋᐦᒡ ᑳ ᒌ ᒦᒋᑦ ᔖᑳᔨᐤ᙮ ᐋᔫᐧᐃᒄ ᓃᔕ ᑳ ᐧᐋᐱᒫᑦ ᑐᔅ ᐋᐦ ᔖᑳᐅᐱᔨᔨᐦᒡᐦ ᐊᐧᐋᔨᐤᐦ᙮

ᐧᐄᒑᐸᑎᔨᒣᐤ ᐧᓰᔅ ᐅᔫ ᐃᔅᐧᑫᐤ ᒣᐧᑳᓐ ᑲᒻᐸᓃᐤ ᐊᑖᐧᐋᑲᒥᑯᐦᒡ ᑳᒌ ᐋᐸᑎᓯᑦ᙮ ᒌ ᐸᔅᑯᐦᐊᒻ ᐊᓂᔫᐦ ᒪᓯᓇᐦᐄᑲᓂᔕ ᐁ ᓅᑯᓂᔨᒡ ᐁ ᐃᑕᒋᐦᑖᑯᓂᔨᒡ ᑫᐧᑳᔫ, ᐊᓂᔫ ᒫᒃ ᐁ ᐃᐦᑎᑦ ᐊᓐ ᐃᔅᐧᑫᐤ ᐁᐅᒄ ᑳᒌ ᐃᐦᑎᑦ ᓈᔅᒡ ᐋᔅᒡ ᐁᒌ ᒥᓂᐦᐧᑫᑦ᙮ ᐯᔭᒄ ᒥᓂᑯᔥ ᓵᔅ ᒦᓐ ᑳᒌ ᒥᓂᐦᐧᑫᑦ᙮ ᐁᑯᓐ ᐱᔑᒄ ᑳᒌ ᐃᐦᑎᑦ ᐃᔅᑲᓂᒌᔑᑳᐤ ᐃᔅᑫᑳ ᒌ ᑌᐱᔑᒨᐧᐋ ᐁ ᐃᐦᑎᑦ᙮ ᒌ ᐧᐋᐸᒣᐤ ᐧᓰᔅ ᐊᓂᔫ ᐃᔅᐧᑫᐤᐦ ᒧᔮᓪ ᐁᐧᐄ ᓴᒋᓯᔨᒡ ᐁ ᐃᔑᓈᑯᓯᔨᒡ, ᒧᐧᐁᐦᒡ ᓂᐹᒌ ᓂᐱᓐ ᐁᑳ ᒥᓂᐦᐧᑫᔮᓄ ᐁ ᐃᑌᔨᐦᑕᒥᔨᒡ, ᐋᑦ ᒫᒃ ᒥᔅᑕᐦᐄ ᓂᐱᔫ ᐁᒌ ᒥᓂᐦᐧᑫᔨᒡ᙮ ᓈᔅᒡ ᑖᐧᐯ ᒌ ᓴᒋᓵᓈᑯᓵ᙮ ᒌ ᐃᐦᑖᐤ ᒦᓐ ᑯᑕᒃ ᐃᔅᐧᑫᐤ ᐊᓂᑕ ᐁ ᐋᐸᑎᓯᑦ ᒌ ᐧᐋᐸᒣᐤ ᑖᓐ ᐁ ᐃᔅᐸᔨᔨᒡ ᐊᓂᔫᐦ ᐃᔅᐧᑫᐤᐦ ᓈᔅᒡ ᐧᐁᑖᒡ ᐁᑳ ᐧᐋᐸᐦᑕᒥᔨᒡ᙮ ᑳ ᐄᑖᑦ ᐊᓂᔫᐦ ᐃᔅᐧᑫᐤᐦ ᓂᑐᐦᑯᐄᓐ ᑫᒌ ᓂᑐᐧᐋᐸᒫᔨᒡ = ᒌ ᐯᐦᑕᒧᑯᐸᓄ ᑮᐹ ᐁ ᐃᐦᑕᑯᓂᔨᒡ ᐋᐦᑯᓯᐧᐃᓂᔫ ᐁ ᐃᐦᑑᑖᑯᑦ ᐊᐧᐁᓐ ᓈᔅᒡ ᑫᒌ ᐹᐦᑯᑖᐦᑕᐦᒃ ᑲᔦ ᐁᑳ ᑫᒌ ᐊᑎ ᐧᐋᐸᐦᑕᐦᒃ᙮ ᒫᔅᑰᒡ ᐃᐦᑕᑯᓂᔨᑫ ᓂᑐᐦᑯᐄᓐ ᑫᒌ ᐧᐄᒋᐦᐋᑲᓅᑦ ᐊᐧᐁᓐ ᐅᔫ ᐁ ᐃᔅᐸᔨᑦ ᒌ ᐃᑌᔨᐦᑕᒻ᙮ ᓇᒧᐃ ᒥᐦᑫᑐ ᒌᔑᑳᐤ ᐊᓂᑌ ᐃᔑ, ᐊᓐ ᐃᔅᐧᑫᐤ ᒨᔥ ᑳ ᐹᐦᑯᑖᐦᑕᐦᒃ ᑳ ᒦᓐ ᒌ ᐯᒋ ᐋᐸᑎᓰ ᐁᒌ ᐊᔮᑦ ᐁ ᒥᔖᔨᒡ ᐸᒋᔥᑲᐦᐄᑲᓂᔫ ᐁ ᐱᐧᔮᐱᔅᑰᓂᔨᒡ ᑲᔦ ᐧᐋᔑᓂᐦᑖᑲᓈᐱᔅᑰᔨᐦᒡ᙮ ᑳ ᐸᒋᔥᑲᐦᐊᐦᒃ ᐴᒑᔑᔫ ᐃᓐᓴᓚᓐ ᐁ ᐃᐦᑕᑯᓂᔨᒡ ᐊᓂᑕ, ᑳ ᓵᑲᔅᒋᓄᐱᑖᑦ ᐊᓂᔫ ᐸᒋᔥᑲᐦᐄᑲᓂᔫ ᐁᒄ ᑳ ᐸᒋᔥᑲᐦᐆᓯᑦ ᐁᐅᒄ ᒫᒃ ᐅᔫ ᑳ ᐃᐦᑎᑦ ᒣᔑᑯᓪ ᒌᔑᑳᐤ᙮ ᒌ ᐃᐧᑌᐤ ᒣᔑᑯᓪ ᒌᔑᑳᐤ ᑫ ᐃᐦᑑᑖᓯᑦ ᐅᔫ ᑫ ᐃᔥᐱᔥ ᐱᒫᑎᓯᐧᑫ᙮ ᐋᔥᑰ ᒫᒃ ᒌ ᓂᑐᐧᐁᔨᐦᑖᑯᓂᔫ ᐁᑎᑑ ᒥᔅᑕᐦᐄ ᑫᒌ ᐃᔥᐱᔥ ᐋᐸᒋᐦᑖᑦ; ᐁ ᒨᔑᐦᑖᑦ ᐁ ᓇᓇᒥᐸᔨᑦ ᒫᒃ ᐁᑯᑦ ᑳᒌ ᒦᒋᑦ ᑫᐧᑳᔫ ᐁ ᒌᑳᐅᓂᔨᒡ᙮ ᐁᐅᒄ

l'époque, et elle avait soif. Elle posa des étiquettes de prix sur une pile de boîtes, puis elle se précipita vers la fontaine, y but une tasse entière d'eau et revint travailler. Une minute plus tard, elle avait besoin de boire à nouveau. Elle but et but, toute la journée, mais ne pouvait étancher sa soif. Rose pouvait voir le désespoir sur son visage, comme si elle allait mourir de soif même après avoir bu autant d'eau, et c'était quelque chose de terrible à voir. Une autre dame qui travaillait là vit tout cela, et remarqua également que la vision de la dame assoiffée avait beaucoup baissé en quelques semaines. Elle dit gentiment dit à la dame assoiffée d'aller chez le médecin; elle avait entendu parler d'une maladie qui donnait soif aux gens et affectait leur vue. Il y avait peut-être un remède. Quelques jours plus tard, la dame assoiffée était de retour au travail avec une énorme seringue en verre et en métal. Elle plantait l'aiguille dans un flacon d'insuline, tirait sur le piston pour remplir la seringue et s'injectait dans la chair tous les jours. Elle devait faire cela, disait-elle, pour le reste de sa vie. Parfois, l'insuline ne suffisait pas; elle se sentait fébrile et courait vers le chariot à café pour se mettre un morceau de sucre dans la bouche. C'était la deuxième personne diabétique que Rose ait jamais rencontré.

she was thirsty. She stuck some price tickets on a stack of boxes, then hustled over to the water fountain, gulped a whole cup of water, and came back to work. One minute later, she needed to drink again. She drank and drank, all day long, but couldn't quench her thirst. Rose could see the desperation on her face, as if she would die of thirst even after having so much water, and it was something terrible. Another lady working there saw all this, and noticed too that the thirsty lady's vision had gotten much worse in a few weeks. She gently told the thirsty lady to go to the doctor – she had heard about an illness that made people thirsty and affected their eyesight. Maybe there was some medicine. A few days later, the thirsty lady was back at work with an enormous glass-and-metal syringe. She stabbed the needle into a bottle of insulin, pulled back to fill the syringe, and injected it into her flesh every single day. She would have to do this, she said, for the rest of her life. Sometimes the insulin wouldn't be enough; she would feel shaky and would run to the coffee tray and pop a sugar cube into her mouth. She was the second person with diabetes that Rose ever met.

ᒨᔮᒼ ᒫᒃ ᓈᔥᒡ ᒋᔥᒋᑯᒡ ᑳ ᐄᔑᓈᑯᐦᒡ ᓈᔥᒡ ᐋᐦ ᐃᔮᔨᐧᒫᐅᐦᐄᐧᐋᒡ ᐋᐦ ᔖᑳᐅᐱᔨᓈᓂᐧᐃᒡ ᐊᓂᑖᐦ ᐃᐦᑖᐧᐃᓂᐦᒡ᙮ ᒉᔅ ᐅᐧᐄᒑᐧᐋᑭᓐᐦ ᑮᔮᐦ ᐊᓂᔮᐦ ᐹᔕᒡ ᑳ ᐧᐄᒋᔨᒡᐦ ᐋᐦ ᐄᑖᒡ, ᒋᔖᔨᔨᐅᒡ ᑮᔮᐦ ᐊᓂᔮᐦ ᐱᔥᒡ ᐅᐧᐋᐦᑯᒫᑭᓐᐦ ᒌᐦ ᔖᑳᐅᐱᔨᔨᐤᐦ᙮ ᒑᒃ ᐹᐦᐹᔨᒄ ᐊᓂᔮᐦ ᓃᐧᔖᔥᒡ ᐋᐦ ᐃᐦᑎᔑᔨᒡᐦ ᐧᐄᒋᔖᓂᐧᑳᒼᐦ ᑳ ᐄᑖᑭᓂᐧᐃᐧᐃᔨᒡᐦ ᐋᐦ ᔖᑳᐅᐱᔨᔨᒡᐦ, ᑮᔮᐦ ᐹᔨᒄ ᐊᓂᔮᐦ ᐧᐋᐧᐋᒡ ᓃᐧᔖᐤ ᐋᐦ ᒌᐦ ᐅᔨᑯᐦᐄᓯᔨᒡᐦ ᐊᐧᐋᔑᔥᐦ ᐋᐦ ᐃᔮᐧᐋᔨᒡᐦ ᐅᐦᒋ ᐊᓂᔮ ᐋᐦ ᒌᐦ ᔖᑳᐅᐱᔨᔨᒡᐦ᙮ ᑳ ᐱᐳᓂᔨᒡ 1991, ᐋᑯᑎᐦ ᑳ ᒋᔅᑖᐱᑎᔩᑦ ᒉᔅ ᐊᓂᑖᐦ ᓂᑐᐦᑯᔨᓈᐱᑎᔩᐧᐃᓂᐦᒡ᙮ ᐊᓂᑖᐦ ᐄᔑ ᐅᑖᐦᒡ ᓃᔥᑎᓂᐧᐋᐱᐳᓐᐦ ᐋᑯᑎᐦ ᑳ ᐧᐄᒑᐱᑎᔩᒫᑦ ᐊᓂᔮᐦ ᐃᔅᐧᑳᐤ ᓈᔥᒡ ᒨᔥ ᑳ ᐹᐦᑯᑖᐦᑎᒥᔨᒡᐦ ᑮᔮᐦ ᓂᔥᑐᒥᑎᓂᐧᐋᐱᐳᓐᐦ ᑳ ᐄᔥᐱᔑ ᐧᐋᐱᒫᑦ ᐊᓂᔮᐦ ᐃᔥᐧᑳᔑᔥᐦ ᑳ ᒌᔥᑎᐦᐅᓯᔨᒡᐦ ᐊᓂᑖᐦ ᒦᔩᐅᑭᒥᑯᐦᒡ ᒫᐧᑳᒡ ᑳ ᒋᔅᑯᑎᒫᓯᑦ ᑳ ᐄᔥᐹᔨᒡ ᒋᔅᑯᑎᒫᑑᑭᒥᑯᐦᒡ, ᐅᔮ ᒫᒃ ᐊᓅᐦᒡ ᐋᔑᑯᒌᔑᑳᐤᐦ ᐧᐋᐧᐄᒋᐦᐋᐤ ᐊᐧᐋᔨᐤᐦ ᐋᐦ ᔖᑳᐅᐱᔨᔨᒡᐦ᙮ ᓈᓈᓂᒌᒼ ᐊᑎ ᒥᐦᒑᑎᐧᐃᒡ ᐊᐧᐋᓂᒌ ᐋᐦ ᔖᑳᐅᐱᔨᒡ = ᑮᔮᐦ ᒑᑳᑦ ᒥᓯᐧᐋ ᓈᔥᒡ ᐋᐦ ᑯᔥᑯᐦᐄᑯᒡ ᐧᐋᐦᑎᒧᐧᐋᑭᓂᐧᐃᐧᑖᐤᐦ᙮

“ᓂᑎᐧᐃ ᓂᑏ ᐃᑎᑭᐧᐃᓈᒑ,” ᐄᑎᑰ ᒫᓐᐦ, “ᑖᐹ ᓂᐦᑖ ᓂᒦᒋᓐ ᒑᐧᑳᓐ ᐋᐦ ᔒᐧᐋᒡ᙮ ᓂᒥᔮᒋᒑ ᐋᐦ ᔖᑳᐅᐱᔨᔮᓐ᙮”

ᒉᔅ ᒫᒃ ᑯᐃᔅᒄ ᐧᐄᐦᒌᒧᐧᐋᐤ, ᐋᐦ ᐄᔨᔨᐅᔨᒥᐦᐋᑦ ᐋᑳ ᑭᔅᑎᐦᐧᐃᔨᒡᐦ ᐊᓂᔮᐦ ᓂᑐᐦᑯᔨᓐᐦ ᑮᔮᐦ ᓂᑐᐦᑯᔨᓂᔅᐧᑳᐤᐦ, ᐊᓂᔮ ᐃᔮᐱᒋᐦᐋᒡ

ᐅᔫᐦ ᓃᔕ ᐊᐧᐁᔫᐦ ᑳ ᒋᔅᑫᔨᒫᑦ ᐧᒉᔅ ᐁ ᐊᔮᔨᒡ ᔩᐧᐋᑲᒥᐦᐧᑫᐅᐋᐦᑯᓯᐧᐃᓂᔫ᙮

ᑫᒃ ᒫ ᓯᔅᒋᑯᒡ ᒌ ᐯᐦᑖᑯᓐ ᐁ ᔩᐧᐋᑲᒥᐦᐧᑳᓅᐦᒡ ᐊᓂᑕ ᐊᐦᑖᐧᐃᓂᐦᒡ᙮ ᐧᒉᔅ ᐅᐧᐄᒉᐧᐋᑲᓐᐦ, ᐅᑑᑌᒼᐦ, ᒥᐦᒉᑐ ᒋᒐᐃᓅᒡ, ᒉᒋᒼ ᐊᓂᑌ ᐁ ᐯᔭᑯᑌᐅᔩᑦ ᒌ ᐃᐦᑖᐅᒡ ᐁ ᔩᐧᐋᑲᒥᐦᐧᑫᐧᑖᐤ᙮ ᐸᐦᐯᔭᒄ ᐧᐄᒋᔖᓐ ᐁ ᐃᔅᐧᑫᐧᐃᔨᒡ ᒌ ᒥᔅᑳᑲᓅᔫ ᐁ ᔩᐧᐋᑲᒥᐦᐧᑫᔨᒡ, ᐯᔭᒄ ᐊᓂᔫᐦ ᓃᐧᔖᐤ ᒌ ᐧᐊᓇᐦᐁᐤ ᐅᑕᐧᐋᔒᒼᐦ ᐊᓂᔫᐦ ᐅᐦᒋ ᐁ ᔩᐧᐋᑲᒥᐦᐧᑫᑦ᙮ 1991 ᑳ ᐃᒋᔥᑌᒡ ᐊᔅᒌᐤ ᐊᒋᐦᑖᓯᓐ ᐁᑯᑦ ᑳ ᒋᐦᒋ ᐊᑐᔅᑯᐧᐋᑦ ᐧᒉᔅ ᒥᔫᐱᒫᑎᔩᐅᓐ ᐊᓈᓈᑲᒋᐦᑖᑲᓅᒡ, ᑳ ᓈᓈᑲᒋᐦᐋᑦ ᑲᔦ ᑳᓇᓂᑐᐧᐋᐸᒫᑦ ᐊᐧᐁᔫᐦ ᔮᑯᐦᓯᔨᒡ ᒌ ᐄᑖᐸᑎᓰ (CHR)᙮ ᓃᔥᑐᓅ ᐱᐳᓐᐦ ᒫᒃ ᒌ ᒦᔮᐅᐸᓂᔫ ᐊᓂᑕ ᑳ ᐅᐦᒋ ᒋᔅᑫᔨᒫᑦ ᐊᓂᔫ ᐃᔅᐧᑫᐤ ᓃᔥᑕᒼ ᑳ ᐧᐄᒑᐸᑎᓰᒫᑦ ᐁᒄ ᓂᔥᑐᒥᑐᓅ ᐱᐳᓐᐦ ᒌ ᒦᔮᐅᐸᔨᓂᔫ ᐊᓂᑕ ᑳ ᐅᐦᒋ ᐧᐋᐸᒫᑦ ᐊᓂᔫᐦ ᐃᔅᑫᔅ ᑳ ᐸᒋᔅᑲᐦᐆᓯᔨᒡ, ᑫᒃ ᒫᒃ ᒌ ᐃᔑᓈᑯᓂᔫ ᑫᒌ ᐧᐄᒋᐦᐋᑦ ᐊᐧᐁᔫᐦ ᑳ ᔩᐧᐋᑲᒥᐦᐧᑫᔨᒡ᙮ ᒉᔑᑯᒼ ᐲᓯᒼ ᒌ ᐃᐦᑑᐅᒡ ᒦᓐ ᑯᑕᑲᒡ ᐁ ᒥᔅᑳᑲᓄᔨᒡ ᐁ ᔩᐧᐋᑲᒥᐦᐧᑫᐧᑖᐤ ᒥᐦᒉᑐ ᒫᒃ ᐅᒌ ᒌ ᑯᔥᑯᐸᔫᒡ ᐁ ᐧᐄᐦᑕᒧᐧᐋᑲᓅᐧᑖᐤ ᐁ ᔩᐧᐋᑲᒥᐦᐧᑫᐧᑖᐤ᙮

ᓇᒧᐃ ᓈᓂᑑ, ᐁ ᐃᑎᑯᑦ, ᓇᒧᐃ ᐧᐄᔅᑳᒡ ᓂᒦᒋᓐ ᑫᐧᑳᓐ ᐁ ᓰᑲᐅᒡ᙮ ᓇᒧᐃ ᓈᓂᑑ ᓂᔩᐧᐋᑲᒥᐦᐧᑫᓈᒉ᙮

ᑳᒌ ᐃᐧᑌᑦ ᑲᔦ ᐊᐧᐁᔫ, ᓂᒧᔖᒥᓈᓐ ᑲᔦ ᓅᐦᑯᒥᓈᓐ ᒌ ᒧᐧᐁᐅᒡ ᐋᐃᐦᑯᓈᐤ ᑲᔦ ᓰᐹᐃᐦ ᓇᒧᐃ ᒫᒃ ᐅᐦᒋ ᔩᐧᐋᑲᒥᐦᐧᑫᐅᒡ᙮

Puis, soudainement, on parlait du diabète partout dans la communauté. Les amis et les voisins de Rose, plusieurs aînés et même sa famille étaient diabétiques. Une à une, les sept sœurs de Rose furent diagnostiquées et l'une d'entre elles fit même deux fausses couches à cause de la maladie. En 1991, Rose commença à travailler comme représentante en santé communautaire (RSC) pour le Conseil cri de la santé et des services sociaux de la Baie James. Vingt années s'étaient écoulées depuis qu'elle avait rencontré la dame assoiffée et trente années depuis qu'elle avait vu la fille à l'aiguille à l'école secondaire, et Rose travaillait désormais tous les jours avec des personnes atteintes de diabète. Chaque mois, de plus en plus de gens étaient diagnostiqués pour la première fois. Presque tous étaient surpris.

« Ce n'est pas possible, lui disaient-ils, je ne mange jamais de sucreries. Ça ne peut pas être le diabète ».

Rose expliquait à chaque personne, en langue crie, que les médecins et les infirmières ne pouvaient pas parler, que

Then, suddenly, talk of diabetes was everywhere in the community. Rose's friends and neighbours, several Elders, even her family had diabetes. One by one, Rose's seven sisters were diagnosed, and one of them even had two miscarriages as a result of the disease. In 1991, Rose began working as a Community Health Representative (CHR) for the Cree Board of Health and Social Services of James Bay. Twenty years had passed since she had met the thirsty lady and thirty years since she had seen the girl with the needle in high school, and now Rose worked every day with people with diabetes. More people were being newly diagnosed every month – and almost every one of them was surprised.

"That can't be right," they would say to her. "I never eat sweets. It can't be diabetes."

Rose would explain to each person, in the Cree language that the doctors and nurses couldn't speak, that the flour

ᐱᐦᐧᑳᔑᑭᓐᐦ ᐋᐦ ᐅᔑᐦᐋᒡ ᐴᒋᓂᔥᐦ ᑭᔮᐦ ᐋᐃᐦᑯᓈᐤᐦ ᐋᑦ ᐊ̈ᑲ ᓰᐅᓯᔩᒡᐦ ᐊᔮᐱᒡ ᐋᐦ ᐄᐦᑎᑯᓂᔨᒡ ᐊᓂᑎᐦ ᔖᑳᔨᐤ᙮

ᐊᐧᑳᑎᑯᑦ ᒫᓐᐦ, “ᓂᒧᔓᒻ ᑭᔮᐦ ᓅᐦᑯᒻ ᒨᔥ ᒌᐦ ᒧᐧᐋᐧᐃᒡ ᐋᐃᐦᑯᓈᐤᐦ ᑭᔮᐦ ᐴᒋᓂᔥᐦ ᓂᒥᒌᔨᐧᐋ ᒫᒃ ᐅᐦᒋ ᔖᑳᐅᐱᔨᔪᐧᐃᒡ ᐧᐄᔨᐧᐋᐤ᙮”

“ᑖᐧᐹᐦ,” ᐄᑖᐤ ᒍᔅ, “ᑭᔨᐧᐹ ᑳ ᒧᐧᐋᒡ ᐋᐃᐦᑯᓈᐤᐦ ᑭᔮᐦ ᐴᒋᓂᔥᐦ᙮ ᒥᑯ ᒫᒃ ᒨᔥ ᒌᐦ ᐃᔮᔭᐦᒌᐧᐃᒡ ᐊᓐ ᒌᔮᓂᐤ ᐊ̈ᑲ ᔖᔥ ᐃᔨᐦᑎᔨᐦᑯ᙮ ᓈᔥᑖᐧᐹᐦ ᐄᔨᐦᒡ ᐄᔑᓈᑯᓐ ᔖᔥ ᐱᒫᑎᓰᐧᐃᓐ ᑳᐹᒋ ᐄᔑᓈᑯᓂᔨᒡ ᓈᑖᐦ ᐧᐄᔨᐧᐋᐤ ᐋᔥᑯ ᐋᐦ ᒌᐦ ᒦᔫᔮᔭᐦᒌᒡ᙮”

ᐊᓂᑖᐦ ᒫᒃ ᐊᔨᒧᐧᐊ̈ᔭᐲᐦᒡ ᑭᔮᐦ ᐊᓂᑖᐦ ᒋᔅᑯᑎᒫᑑᑭᒥᑯᐦᒡ ᐋᑯᑖᐦ ᑳ ᐄᑐᐦᑖᑦ ᐋᐦ ᒋᔅᑯᑎᒫᒑᑦ ᑭᔮᐦ ᐋᐦ ᐃᔮᔭᒧᑎᐦᒃ ᐋᐦ ᔖᑳᐅᐱᔨᓈᓂᐧᐃᐧᐃᔨᒡ, ᑭᔮᐦ ᐋᐦ ᐧᐄᐦᑎᒧᐧᐋᑦ ᐊᐧᐋᔨᐤᐦ ᑖᐱᔥᑯᓐ ᐅᔥᐧᑳᔥᐦ ᑭᔮᐦ ᐱᑖᑎᔅᐦ ᐋᐦ ᐄᐦᑎᑯᓂᔨᒡ ᔖᑳᔨᐤ, ᑭᔮᐦ ᐋᐦ ᐧᐄᐦᑎᒧᐧᐋᑦ ᓈᐅᔥ ᐋᐦ ᐱᐹᒧᐦᑖᑦ ᐊᐧᐋᓐ ᓃᔓᒌᔑᑳᐤᐦ ᒋᑭ ᒌᐦ ᓃᔑᐱᔨᔨᐤ ᔖᑳᔨᐤ ᐅᒥᐦᑯᐦᒡ, ᒥᓂᐦᐧᑳᐧᐃᓂᐦᒡ ᐋᑯᑎᐦ ᑭᔮᐦ ᐋᐦ ᐃᐦᑎᑯᐦᒡ ᔖᑳᐤ ᐋᑦ ᐊ̈ᑲ ᔒᐧᐋᑭᒥᒡ, ᐅᓵᒻ ᐋᐦ ᐃᔮᔭᒫᔭᐦᑎᒃ ᐊᐧᐋᓐ ᐋᑯᑎᐦ ᑭᔮᐦ ᒐ ᒌᐦ ᐅᐦᒋ ᐄᔅᑯᐱᔨᔨᒡ ᐅᔖᑲᒻ᙮ ᐊᔮᐱᒡ ᒫᒃ ᒫᐧᑲᒡ ᓈᓈᓂᒌᒻ ᐊᑎ ᒥᐦᒐᑎᐧᐃᒡ ᐊᐧᐋᓂᒌ ᐋᐦ ᔖᑳᐅᐱᔨᔨᒡ ᑭᔮᐦ ᑯᑎᒋᔨᐤ ᐋᐦᑯᓯᐧᐃᓂᔨᐤ ᐋᐦ ᐅᑎᐦᑎᑯᒡ ᓂᒥ ᐅᐦᒋ ᐄᔥᐱᔒᐤ ᒍᔅ ᒐᒃ ᐋᑯᐦ ᑳ ᐅᑎᓈᑭᓂᐧᐃᐧᐃᔨᒡᐦ ᒦᓐ ᐊᐧᐋᔨᐤᐦ ᒐ ᐧᐄᒋᐦᐄᑯᑦ ᑭᔨᐧᐹ ᐋᐦ ᒌᐦ

ᐁᑯ ᑳᒌ ᐄᑖᑦ ᐊᓂᔫ ᐁ ᐃᑎᑯᑦ, ᐁᐦᐁ ᑖᐧᐯ ᒌ ᒧᐧᐁᐅᒡ ᐋᐊᐦᑯᓈᐤ ᑲᔦ ᓰᐹᐃᐦ᙮

ᒥᑯ ᒫᒃ ᒨᔥ ᐧᐁᓯᓐ ᒌ ᐊ̈ᔭᐦᒌᐅᒡ ᐁᑳ ᐃᐦᑎᔮᐦᑯ ᒋᔮᓅ ᓵᔅ᙮ ᐋᐦᒌᐤ ᒋᑎᐦᑎᓈᓅ ᐊᓐᒌᔥ ᑖᓐ ᑳ ᐯᒋ ᐃᐦᑎᐧᑖᐤ ᐧᐄᐧᐋᐤ᙮

ᒌ ᐊᔨᒨ ᒫᓐᐦ ᐊᔨᒧ̈ᔭᐲᐦᒡ ᑲᔦ ᐊᓂᑌ ᒋᔅᑯᑕᒫᒉᐅᑲᒥᑯᐦᒡ ᐁ ᐋᔨᒨᑕᐦᒃ ᐁ ᓯ̈ᑲᐅᐸᔨᓈᓄᔨᒡ ᐁ ᓰᐦᒋᒫᑦ ᐊᐧᐁᔫᐦ ᐁᑳ ᑖᐱᔅᑯᓐ ᐧᐋᐸᔫᒥᓂᔅ ᑲᔦ ᐸᑌᑎᔅ ᑫᒌ ᒥᒋᔨᒡ ᐯᔭᐧᑳᐤ ᐁ ᒦᒋᓯᔨᒡ ᐧᐁᔥ ᑖᐱᔥᑯᓐ ᐅᔫᐦ ᓯ̈ᑲᐅᓐ, ᑲᔦ ᒌ ᐃᑌᐤ ᑫ ᐧᐄᒋᐦᐄᑯᑦ ᐊᐧᐁᓐ ᒋᓅᐅᔥ ᐁ ᐱᒧᐦᑌᑦ ᐧᐁᔅ ᐁᑯᑦ ᑫ ᐅᐦᒋ ᐋᔑᐸᔨᒡ ᐅᔖᑳᒻ ᐧᐃᔦᔅ ᓃᔓ ᒌᔑᑳᐤ ᐧᐄᒋᐦᐄᐧᐁᐸᔫ, ᑲᔦ ᑳ ᒥᔅᑯᐧᐋᑲᒥᐦᒡ ᒥᓂᐦᐧᑫᐧᐃᓐ ᒥᔅᑕᐦᐄ ᐁ ᐃᐦᑕᑯᐦᒡ ᐊᓂᑕ ᔖᑳᐤ ᐋᑦ ᐁᑳ ᓰᐧᐋᑲᒥᐦᒡ ᐁ ᐃᔅᐸᑯᐦᒡ, ᑲᔦ ᒫᒃ ᐊᐧᐁᓐ ᒨᔥ ᑳ ᐋᔨᒣᔨᐦᑕᐦᒃ ᐋᐦᒡ ᓇᒧᐃ ᒋᑲ ᐅᐦᒋ ᒥᔫᐸᔫ ᐁ ᓰᐧᐋᑲᒥᐦᐧᑫᑦ᙮ ᐋᑦ ᒫᒃ ᐅᔫ ᐁᒌ ᐃᐦᑎᑦ, ᔮᐸᒡ ᒌ ᐊᑎ ᑯᑕᑲᒡ ᐊᐧᐁᓂᒌ ᐁ ᒥᔅᑳᑲᓄᔨᒡ ᐁ ᓰᐧᐋᑲᒥᐦᐧᑫᐧᑖᐤ ᑲᔦ ᑯᑕᒃ ᐋᐦᑯᓯᐧᐃᓐᐦ ᐁ ᐊᔩᐧᑖᐤ ᑫᒃ ᓇᒧᐃ ᐅᐦᒌ ᐃᐦᑑ ᐧᓵᔅ ᑫᒌ

la farine des boulettes de pâte et de la bannique n'avait peut-être pas un goût sucré, mais qu'il s'agissait néanmoins d'une sorte de sucre.

« Mais, disaient-ils, nos grands-parents mangeaient de la bannique et des boulettes de pâte et ils ne faisaient pas de diabète ».

« Oui, répondait Rose, ils mangeaient de la bannique et des boulettes de pâte. Mais pensez à tout l'exercice qu'ils faisaient et que nous ne faisons pas. Pensez à toutes les façons dont nos vies sont différentes des leurs ».

Elle commença à parler du diabète à la radio et dans les écoles, à enseigner aux gens à ne pas manger du riz et des pommes de terre dans le même repas parce que les deux sont une sorte de sucre, à enseigner qu'une longue marche pouvait faire baisser la glycémie pendant jusque deux jours, à enseigner que l'alcool pouvait être dense en sucre même s'il ne goûtait pas sucré, à enseigner que le stress aggravait la maladie. Et pourtant, il y avait tellement de nouveaux diagnostics de diabète et d'autres maladies chroniques que Rose ne pouvait pas faire tout le travail elle-même et que le Conseil cri de la santé dut embaucher

in dumplings and bannock might not taste sweet, but it was a kind of sugar nevertheless.

"But," they would say, "our grandparents ate bannock and dumplings and they didn't have diabetes."

"Yes," Rose would answer, "they ate bannock and dumplings. But think of all the exercise they did that we don't do. Think of all the ways our lives are different from theirs."

She began talking about diabetes on the radio and in schools, teaching people not to have both rice and potatoes in the same meal because both are a kind of sugar, teaching that a long walk would lower blood sugar for up to two days, teaching that alcohol could be dense with sugar even if it didn't taste sweet, teaching that stress aggravated the disease. And still, there were so many new diagnoses of diabetes and other chronic illnesses that Rose couldn't do all the work herself and the Cree Board of Health had to hire another CHR for Chisasibi just to meet the demand.

ᐊᑎᒥᐦᒑᑎᔨᒡᐦ ᐊᐧᐋᔨᐤᐦ ᐋᐦ ᔒᑳᐅᐱᔨᔨᒡᐦ᙮

ᒌᒃ ᒦᓐ ᑯᑎᒃ ᐊᐧᐋᓐ ᑳ ᐅᑎᓈᑭᓂᐧᐃᑦ, ᒦᓐ ᐹᑎᒫᐦ ᒦᓐ ᑯᑎᒃ ᐊᐧᐋᓐ᙮

ᓂᔩᓂᑯᑑᓐᐦ ᑳ ᓂᑑᑎᐹᔨᐦᑎᐦᒃ ᑭᔩᐦ ᐧᐄᔨ ᔪᔅ ᐅᒥᐦᒄ ᐋᐦ ᐋᐱᒥᐦᑖᑦ ᐊᓂᔩᐦ ᒫᔨᐧᐋᑦ ᐊᓂᑖᐦ ᐋᐦ ᐋᐱᑎᔩᑦ ᑳ ᐋᐱᒥᐦᑖᑭᓂᐧᐃᐧᐃᔨᒡᐦ᙮ ᐋᑎᐧᐄ ᓂᒥ ᐅᐦᒋ ᐃᔩᐤ ᐋᐦ ᔒᑳᐅᐱᔨᓈᓂᐧᐃᐧᐃᔨᒡ, ᒥᒄ ᒫᒃ ᐊᓂᑖᐦ ᐋᐦ ᐹᔨᑯᑖᐅᔩᒡ ᐋᑯᑎᐦ ᑳ ᐃᔩᔨᒡᐦ ᐊᐧᐋᔨᐤᐦ ᒫᐧᑳᒡ ᑭᔨᐧᐹ ᓈᔥᒡ ᐋᒃ ᐅᐦᒋ ᒥᒥᔮᐱᔨᔨᒡ ᒑᐧᑳᔩᐤ ᐊᓂᑖᐦ ᐧᐄᒋᐦᐧᐋᐦᒡ, ᐋᐦᐧᒫᔩᐦ ᐅᐦᒋ ᐳᓃᒡᐦ ᐅᓈᐹᒻᐦ ᐋᐦ ᒥᓂᐦᐧᐋᔨᒡᐦ᙮ ᓈᔥᒡ ᒥᐦᒑᑐ ᐊᐧᐋᓂᒌ ᐊᓂᑎᐦ ᐃᐦᑖᐧᐃᓂᐦᒡ ᐋᐦ ᒌᐦ ᐋᐦᑯᓯᒡ᙮ ᐋᑎᐧᐄ ᑭᔨᐧᐹ ᒥᐦᒑᑐᐱᐳᓐᐦ ᓂᒥ ᐅᐦᒋ ᐧᐃᔩᔥᑎᐤ ᔪᔅ ᓈᑑᑎᐹᔨᐦᑎᐦᒃ ᐊᓂᔩ ᐅᒥᐦᒄ᙮ ᒥᐦᒑᑐᐱᐳᓐᐦ ᒌᒃ ᒌᐦ ᒌᐧᐋᐦᑎᑖᐤ ᐊᓂᑖᐦ ᐧᐄᒋᐧᐋᐦᒡ ᒑ ᒌᐦ ᓂᑑᑎᐹᔨᒫᑦ ᐊᐧᐋᔨᐤᐦ ᐊᓂᑎᐦ ᐋᐦ ᐹᔨᑯᑖᐅᔩᒡ, ᐅᓈᐹᒻᐦ ᑭᔩᐦ ᐅᑎᐧᐋᔑᔒᒻᐦ᙮ ᒌᒃ ᑳ ᐃᐦᑐᑎᐦᒃ ᐊᓂᔩ ᒑᐧᑳᔩᐤ ᑳ ᐄᑖᔨᐦᑎᐦᒃ ᐋᒃ ᓂᐦᑖ ᒐ ᐃᐦᑐᑎᐦᒃ ᐋᔮᐧᐃᒄ ᒐ ᐊᔑᒫᑦ ᐅᑎᐧᐋᔑᔒᒻᐦ ᐱᐧᑫᑭᑖ ᑳ ᐄᔑᓂᐦᑳᑖᔨᒡ = ᒥᒄ ᑭᔨᐧᐹ ᐋᒃ ᐅᐦᒋ ᐃᐦᑐᑎᐧᐋᑦ ᐊᓂᔩ ᑳ ᐃᐦᑐᑎᐧᐋᑭᓂᐧᐃᑦ ᐊᓂᑖᐦ ᐧᐄᔨ ᒋᔅᑯᑎᒫᑑᑭᒥᑯᐦᒡ ᑳ ᐃᐦᑖᑦ᙮

ᐹᔨ··ᑳᐤ ᒫᒃ ᐋᐦ ᒌᔑᑳᔨᒡ, 1997 ᑳ ᐄᒋᔥᑖᔨᒡ ᐋᐦ ᐱᐳᓂᔨᒡ, ᐄᔨᐦᒡ ᑳ ᐄᔅᐱᔨᔨᒡ ᐋᐦ ᓂᑑᑎᐹᔨᐦᑎᐦᒃ ᐅᒥᐦᒄ: ᒑᑲᑦ ᔒᔥ ᐋᐦ ᐃᔩᑦ

ᐯᔨᐧᑳᐸᑎᓯᑦ ᐁ ᐊᑐᔅᑯᐧᐋᑦ ᒥᔮᐱᒫᑎᓰᐅᓐ ᐁᓈᓈᑲᒋᐦᑖᑲᓅᒡ ᐁᒄ ᒦᓐ ᑯᑕᒃ ᐊᐧᐁᓐ ᑳ ᐅᑖᔅᑯᓈᑲᓅᑦ ᒉᒌ ᐧᐄᒐᐸᑎᓰᒥᑯᑦ ᐧᑫᔅ ᐊᓂᑕ ᒋᓵᓰᐲᐦᒡ᙮

ᒉᒃ ᒦᓐ ᑯᑕᒃ ᐊᐧᐁᓐ ᒌ ᐅᑖᔅᑯᓈᑲᓅ᙮

ᐁᒄ ᒦᓐ ᑯᑕᒃ ᑳ ᐅᑖᔅᑯᓈᑲᓅᑦ᙮

ᓂᔩᓂᑯᑌᐦᒡ ᒫᒃ ᒌ ᓂᑑ ᒋᔅᑫᒥᓰ ᐧᑫᔅ ᐁ ᓂᑑ ᒋᔅᑫᔨᑕᐦᒃ ᑲᔦ ᐧᐄ ᐅᒥᐦᒄ ᑖᓐ ᐁ ᐃᔥᐱᔥ ᔒᑳᐅᓂᔨᔨᒡ᙮ ᒌ ᐊᔩᐤ ᐊᓂᔮ ᔩᐸᒋᐦᑖᑦ ᐊᐧᐁᓐ ᐅᔮ ᐁ ᐃᔑ ᓂᑑ ᒋᔅᑫᔨᒥᓯᑦ᙮ ᓇᒧᐃ ᑮᐸ ᐅᐦᒋ ᓰᐧᐋᑲᒥᐦᐧᑫᐤ ᐧᐄᔨ ᒥᒄ ᒫᒃ ᐊᓂᑕ ᐁ ᐯᔨᑯᑌᐅᓯᑦ ᒌ ᐃᐦᑖᔮ ᐊᐧᐁᔮᐦ ᐁ ᓰᐧᐋᑲᒥᐦᐧᑫᔨᒡ ᓈᔅᒡ ᒫᒃ ᒌ ᒥᑯᔥᑳᑌᔨᐦᑕᒥᐦᐄᑯᒡ ᐆᔮ ᐊᓂᑕ ᐁᔅᒄ ᒉᐧᑳᒡ ᐁᒌ ᒥᓂᐦᐧᑫᔨᒡ ᐅᓈᐯᓐ᙮ ᒌ ᒥᐦᒉᑎᔮᐦ ᐊᐧᐁᓂᔮᐦ ᐊᓂᑕ ᐅᑎᐦᑖᐧᐃᓂᐧᐋᐦᒡ ᐁᐧᐄ ᐋᐦᑯᓰᐧᐁᔨᐦᑖᑯᓯᔨᒡ᙮ ᒥᐦᒉᑐ ᐱᐳᓐᐦ ᒎᔥ ᐁᑯᓐ ᑳᒌ ᐃᐦᑎᑦ ᐁᓂᑑ ᒋᔅᑫᔨᐦᑕᐦᒃ ᐅᒥᐦᒄ ᐋᑦ ᐁᑳ ᐅᐦᒋ ᓰᐧᐋᑲᒥᐦᐧᑫᑦ᙮ ᐁᑯᓐ ᑳᒌ ᐃᐦᑑᑐᐧᐋᑦ ᑲᔦ ᐅᑕᐧᐋᔑᔒᒻ ᑲᔦ ᐅᓈᐯᒻ᙮ ᒌ ᐃᐦᑑᑕᒻ ᑲᔦ ᐊᓂᔮ ᑳ ᐄᐧᑌᑦ ᐁᑳ ᐧᐄᔅᑳᒡ ᒉ ᐅᐦᒋ ᐃᐦᑎᑦ: ᒌ ᓰᐦᒋᒉᐤ ᐅᑕᐧᐋᔑᔒᒻᐦ ᒉᒌ ᒦᒋᔨᒡ ᐸᐧᑫᑲᑖ = ᒥᒄ ᒌ ᓇᓈᑲᒋᐦᑖᐤ ᐁᑳ ᒉᒌ ᐃᐦᑑᑐᐧᐋᑦ ᑖᓐ ᑳ ᐃᐦᑑᑐᐧᐋᑲᓅᑦ ᐧᐄᔨ ᐊᓂᑌ ᔒᐧᐊᓂᐦᒡ ᑳᒌ ᑲᓇᐧᐁᔨᒫᑲᓅᑦ ᐁ ᒋᔅᑯᑕᒫᓯᑦ᙮

ᐯᔨᐧᑳᐤ 1997 ᐊᓂᑕ ᑳ ᐃᒋᔥᑌᒡ ᐊᔅᒌᐤ ᐊᒋᐦᑖᓯᓐ ᐋᐦᒌᐅᐦ ᒌ ᐃᔅᐸᔨᓂᔮ ᐁ ᓂᑑ ᒋᔅᑫᔨᐦᑕᐦᒃ ᐅᒥᐦᒄ: ᒌ ᓅᑯᓂᔮ ᐊᐱᔒᔥ ᐁᐧᐄ

un autre RSC pour Chisasibi juste pour répondre à la demande.

Et puis un autre.

Et puis un autre.

De temps à autre, Rose utilisait les trousses de test de glycémie pour se dépister elle-même. Elle n'avait pas de symptômes du diabète, mais il c'était un problème commun dans sa famille et elle subissait beaucoup de stress à la maison à cette époque, avant que son mari ne cesse de boire. Tant de gens dans la communauté tombaient malades. Pendant des années, les résultats de ses tests ont été bons, mais Rose a continué à se faire dépister elle-même. Pendant des années, elle a rapporta à la maison des trousses de dépistage du travail et faisait passer des tests à son mari et à tous ses enfants. Elle fit même ce qu'elle s'était juré de ne jamais faire : elle fit manger du brocoli à ses enfants – toutefois, sans jamais utiliser une seule fois les méthodes extrêmes des pensionnats.

Un jour, en 1997, son auto-dépistage révéla un nouveau résultat : pré-diabète, un signe avant-coureur que le diabète

And then another.

And then another.

From time to time, Rose used the glucose-testing kits to screen herself. She didn't have diabetes symptoms, but it ran in her family and there was quite a bit of stress in her home in those days, before her husband stopped drinking. So many people in the community were getting sick. For years her test results were fine but Rose continued self-screening. For years, she brought test kits home from work and tested her husband and all her kids. She even did what she had vowed never to do: she made her children eat broccoli – but without even once using the extreme residential school methods.

One day, in '97, her self-screening showed a new result: pre-diabetes, a warning sign that diabetes was not far away. Rose

ᑳ ᐙᑳᐅᐱᔨᓈᓂᐧᐃᐧᐃᔨᒡ, ᒑ ᒌᐦ ᐄᔑᓈᑯᓂᔨᒡ ᑭᔨᐧᐹ ᒑ ᒌᐦ ᐋᔫᑦ ᐊᓂᔫ ᐋᐦᑯᓯᐧᐃᓂᔨᐤ᙮ ᒑᒃ ᑳ ᒥᔫᑭᓂᐧᐃᑦ ᓂᑐᐦᑯᔨᓂᔨᐤ ᒑ ᐋᐱᒥᐦᑖᑦ ᑭᔫᐦ ᑳ ᐧᐄᐦ ᓈᑭᑎᐧᐋᔨᐦᑎᐦᒃ ᐊᑎᑎᐤ ᒑ ᐙᐙᐧᐄᑦ ᑭᔫᐦ ᑯᐃᔅᒄ ᒑ ᐄᔑ ᒦᒋᓯᑦ᙮ ᐹᔨᐧᑳᐤ ᒫᒃ ᓈᔥᒡ ᐋᐦ ᒥᔦᒑᒋᐙᐹᔫᔨᒡ 2002 ᑳ ᒋᔥᑖᔨᒡ ᐋᐦ ᐱᐳᓂᔨᒡ ᑳ ᐄᑐᐦᑖᑦ ᐊᓂᑖᐦ ᒦᓰᑭᒥᑯᐦᒡ, ᐋᑎ ᐄᔅᑯᐱᑖᑦ ᐊᓂᔫᐦ ᐅᐲᒌᓯᒻᐦ ᒑᔅᒋᓯᑦ ᐊᓂᑖᐦ ᐄᔑ ᐅᑖᐦᒡ ᒥᑖᐦᑐ ᒥᓂᑯᔥ ᐋᐦ ᒌᐦ ᐴᐴᔑᑦ᙮ ᓂᒥ ᓰᐦᒃ ᓈᐅᔥ ᒦᓐ ᒧᔑᐦᑖᑦ ᐋᐦ ᐧᐄᐦ ᐴᐴᔑᑦ᙮ ᐊᓂᑖᐦ ᐋᐦ ᐋᐱᑎᓲᑦ ᐧᐋᑎᓂᐦᒃ ᐊᓂᔫ ᐹᔨᒄ ᐋᐦ ᓂᑑᑎᐹᔨᐦᑎᑭᓂᐧᐃᐧᐃᔨᒡ ᐊᐧᐋᔨᐤᐦ ᐅᒥᐦᑯᔨᐤ᙮ ᒑᔥᑖᐦᒃ ᐊᓂᔫ ᐹᔨᒄ ᐅᑎᐦᒌ, ᐊᓂᑖᐦ ᐋᔑ ᑖᐦᒋᐦᑖᑦ ᐊᓂᑎᐦ ᑳᐙᑯᐦᐄᑭᓃᐧᐃᐧᐃᔑᔨᒡ ᐊᓂᑖᐦ ᐋᔑ ᐲᐦᑖᐦᒃ᙮ ᑳᓂᐧᐋᐱᐦᑎᐦᒃ ᐊᓂᔫ ᐊᒋᔅᑖᓯᓂᔨᐤ ᓈᔥᒡ ᐄᔥᐱᒥᐦᒡ ᐋᐦ ᐄᐦᑎᑯᓂᔨᒡ᙮ ᕈᔅ ᓯᐧᐋᓄ, ᐧᒫᐦᒡ ᐊᓂᔫᐦ ᐃᔥᐧᑳᔑᔥᐦ ᑳ ᐧᐋᐱᒫᑦ ᐋᐦ ᒌᔥᑎᐦᐅᓯᔨᒡᐦ ᐊᓂᑖ ᑳ ᐄᔥᐹᔨᒡ ᒋᔅᑯᑎᒫᑑᑭᒥᑯᐦᒡ ᑳ ᐃᐦᑖᑦ ᑭᔫᐦ ᐊᓂᔫᐦ ᐃᔅᐧᑳᐤᐦ ᑳ ᐧᐄᒐᐱᑎᓲᒪᑦ ᐊᓂᑖᐦ ᐊᑖᐧᐋᐅᑭᒥᑯᐦᒡ, ᐧᒫᐦᒡ ᑭᔫᐦ ᐊᓂᔫᐦ ᒥᓯᐧᐋ ᐧᐄᒋᐙᓂᔥᐦ, ᐋᔨᐧᐃᒄ ᑭᔫᐦ ᐋ ᐃᔫᑦ, ᐋᐦ ᐙᑳᐅᐱᔨᓈᓂᐧᐃᐧᐃᔨᒡ᙮

ᓈᔥᒡ ᐋᐦ ᐲᔑᔫᐦᔫᑦ ᑭᔫᐦ ᒦᓐ ᐊᓂᑖᐦ ᒦᓰᐅᑮᒥᑯᐦᒡ ᐋᔅᐱᐦᑖᑦ᙮

ᐋᔥᒄ ᒫᒃ ᐊᓂᑖᐦ ᓂᑐᐦᑯᔨᓈᐱᑎᓲᐧᐃᓂᐦᒡ ᐋᑯᑖᐦ ᐋᔑ ᐋᐱᑎᓲᑦ ᕈᔅ ᐊᓂᑖᐦ ᒋᔅᓲᐲᐦᒡ, ᓈᐅᔨᐤᐦ ᒫᒃ ᑯᑎᒃᐦ ᐊᐧᐋᔨᐤᐦ ᐧᐋᒋᐦᐄᑯᑦ᙮ ᐋᔨᐧᐃᒄ ᐊᓂᔫ ᐃᔫᐱᑎᔑᔥᑎᐦᒃ ᐋᐦ ᐙᑳᐅᐱᔨᓈᓂᐧᐃᐧᐃᔨᒡ ᑭᔫᐦ ᐋᔨᐧᐃᒄ

ᐙᑳᐅᐸᔨᑦ᙮ ᒌ ᐅᑎᓇᒻ ᐊᓂᔮᐦ ᓂᑐᐦᑯᐄᓐ ᒫᔫᑲᓅᑦ ᐊᐧᐁᓐ ᐁ ᐙᑳᐅᐸᔨᑦ ᑲᔦ ᐁᑎᑑ ᒨᔥ ᒌ ᓴᓵᐅᐸᔨᐦᐆ ᑲᔦ ᒌ ᐁᑎᑑ ᒌ ᓇᓈᑲᒋᐦᑖᐤ ᐁ ᐃᔑ ᒦᒋᓯᑦ᙮ ᐁᒄ ᒦᓐ ᐯᔨᐧᑳᐤ ᐁ ᒥᔮᒌᔑᑲᔑᔨᒡ 2002 ᑳ ᐃᒋᔥᑌᔨᒡ ᐊᔅᒌᐤ ᐊᒋᐦᑖᓯᓂᔮ ᒦᔫᐅᑲᒥᑯᐦᒡ ᒌ ᐃᑐᐦᑌᐤ ᐁᑯᑦ ᑳ ᐅᐦᒋ ᒥᔅᑳᑎᓯᑦ ᒥᑖᐦᑐ ᒥᓂᑯᔥ ᐊᓂᑌ ᐁᒌ ᓯᒋᑦ = ᐁᒄ ᒦᓐ ᔫᐸᒡ ᒥᑖᐦᑐ ᒥᓂᑯᔥ ᐊᓂᑌ᙮ ᔫᔅ ᔫᐸᒡ ᒌᐧᐄ ᒨᔑᐦᑖᐤ ᒦᓐ ᐁᐧᐄ ᓯᒋᑦ᙮ ᑳ ᓂᑐᐧᐋᐦᑕᐦᒃ ᐊᓂᔮ ᔫᐸᑕᓂᔨᒡ ᐊᐧᐁᓐ ᐁ ᓂᑑ ᒋᔅᑫᔨᐦᑕᐦᒃ ᐅᒥᐦᒄ ᑖᓂᑕ ᐁ ᐃᐦᑕᑯᓂᔨᒡ᙮ ᑳ ᐸᒋᔥᑲᐦᐊᔑᑦ ᐅᔨᑭᑎᐦᒐᓂᔥ ᑳ ᐱᒋᑰᓇᐦᒃ ᐅᒥᐦᒄ ᐊᓂᑕ ᐊᓂᔮ ᑳ ᒪᔅᑯᐧᐁᑲᔑᔨᒡ ᐁᒄ ᑳ ᐲᐦᑕᐦᒃ ᐊᓂᑕ ᐹᐦᑕᐦᐄᑲᓄᔨᒡ᙮ ᒌ ᓅᑯᓂᔮ ᐊᒋᐦᑖᓯᓂᔮ, ᒥᔅᑕᐦᐄ ᒌ ᐃᔅᐧᑳᐦᒋᐸᔨᓂᔮ ᐅᐙᑳᒻ᙮ ᐁᐅᑰ ᐧᓵᔅ ᓯᐧᐋᐧᒐ, ᒍᐧᐁᐦᒡ ᐊᓂᔮ ᐃᔅᐧᑫᔅ ᑳᒌ ᐸᒋᔅᑲᐦᐆᓯᔨᒡ ᐊᓂᑌ ᑳᒌ ᒋᔅᑯᑕᒫᓯᐧᒑᐤ ᑲᔦ ᐊᓂᔮ ᐃᔅᐧᑫᐤ ᒨᔥ ᑳᒌ ᐹᐦᑯᒑᐦᑕᒥᔨᒡ ᐦᐋᑦᓯᓐ ᐯᐃ ᑲᒪᐸᓃ ᐊᑖᐧᐋᐅᑲᒥᑯᐦᒡ ᑳᒌ ᐋᐸᑎᓯᑦ, ᑲᔦ ᒥᓯᐧᐁ ᐅᒥᐙ ᐧᓵᔅ, ᐁᒄ ᑲᔦ ᑲᔦ ᐧᐄᔨ ᑳ ᐅᑎᐦᑕᐦᐆᑯᑦ ᐁ ᓃᐧᐋᑲᒥᐦᐧᑳᓄᔨᒡ᙮

ᒌ ᐃᔅᑯᑖᒍ ᐁᒄ ᑳ ᓃᐦᑕᑖᒍᑦ᙮ ᐁᒄ ᒦᓐ ᑳᐤ ᒦᔫᐅᑲᒥᑯᐦᒡ ᑳ ᐃᔅᐸᐦᑖᑦ᙮

ᐁᔅᒄ ᒉᐧᑳᒡ ᐁᐅᒄ ᐁ ᐄᑖᐸᑎᓯᑦ ᐧᓵᔅ ᐁ ᓇᓈᑲᒋᐦᐋᑦ ᐊᐧᐁᔮᐦ ᐊᓂᑕᐦ ᒋᔅᓲᐱᐦᒡ ᒍᐅᔮᐦ ᒫᒍ ᐊᓂᔮ ᐊᐧᐁᔮ ᐧᐋᒐᐸᑎᓲᒥᑯᑦ᙮ ᑳ ᓲᐧᐋᑲᒥᐦᐧᑫᔭᐧᒑᐤ ᓈᓈᑲᒋᐦᐁᐤ ᐧᐄᔨ ᐅᐙ ᒫᒃ ᐁ ᒋᔅᑯᑕᒍᐧᐋᑦ ᐊᐧᐁᔮᐦ ᐁᐅᒄ ᐁ ᐄᑖᐸᑎᓯᑦ,

n'était pas loin. Rose commença à prendre des médicaments et devint encore plus assidue au sujet de l'exercice et de l'alimentation équilibrée. Puis, par une journée ensoleillée du printemps 2002, elle alla aux toilettes au travail et se souvint, en remontant son pantalon, qu'elle était allée à la salle de bain dix minutes plus tôt, et dix minutes avant cela. Elle sentait déjà qu'elle aurait à nouveau besoin de la salle de bain quelques minutes plus tard. Elle traversa le bureau jusqu'à l'armoire contenant les kits de test. Elle se piqua le doigt avec la lancette, essuya le sang sur la bandelette et l'inséra dans le lecteur. Le nombre sur le lecteur de glucose était trop élevé. Rose Swallow, tout comme la fille à la seringue à l'école secondaire et la dame assoiffée du magasin de la Baie d'Hudson, tout comme chacune de ses sœurs, était diabétique.

Elle prit une profonde inspiration et expira. Et puis elle se précipita à nouveau vers la salle de bain.

Rose est toujours une RSC à Chisasibi, avec quatre autres RSC. Elle est responsable du dossier du diabète et passe la majeure partie de son temps de travail à enseigner aux gens, dans

began to take medication and became still more diligent about exercise and careful eating. Then, on a sunny day in spring 2002, she went to the bathroom at work and remembered, as she zipped up her pants, that she had been to the bathroom just ten minutes earlier - and ten minutes before that. She could already feel she would need the toilet in a few minutes again. She crossed the office to the cupboard with the test kits. She pricked her finger with the lancet, wiped the blood on the strip, and inserted it into the reader. The number in the glucose reader was too high. Rose Swallow, like the needle girl in high school and the thirsty lady from the Hudson's Bay Store, like every one of her sisters, had diabetes.

She sucked in a deep breath and let it out. And then she ran back to the bathroom.

Rose is still a CHR in Chisasibi, along with four other CHRs. She's in charge of the diabetes portfolio and spends most of her work time teaching people, in their own language, how to manage the

ᐅᓵ ᐋᑖᐱᑎᓰᑦ ᐋᐦ ᒋᔅᑯᑎᒫᒑᑦ,
ᐄᔮᔮᐅᔮᒧᐧᐃᓂᔮᐤ ᐋᐦ ᐋᐱᒋᔥᑖᑦ, ᐊᓂᑖᐦ
ᒑ ᐄᔑ ᓈᓈᑭᒋᐦᐄᓯᔮᒡᐦ ᐊᐧᐋᔮᐤᐦ ᐋᐦ
ᐙᑳᐅᐱᔮᔮᒡᐦ᙮ ᐆ ᒫᒃ ᐊᓅᐦᒡ ᒑᑲᑦ ᒥᓯᐧᐋ ᐋᐦ
ᐋᑎ ᐱᐹᔮᑯᑖᐅᓰᒡ ᐊᐧᐋᓂᒌ ᑖᐦᑭᐦᐅᑯᐧᐃᒡ
ᐋᐦ ᐙᑳᐅᐱᔮᓈᐧᓂᐧᐃᐧᐄᔮᒡ ᑭᔫᐦ ᓈᓈᓂᒌᒻ
ᐊᑎ ᐊᐧᐋᔑᔒᐅᐧᐃᒡ ᐊᓂᒌ ᐊᐧᐋᓂᒌ
ᐋᑎ ᐃᔫᒡ ᐅᔫ ᐋᐦᑯᓯᐧᐄᓂᔮᐤ᙮ ᐋᔨᐧᐃᒄ
ᐧᐋᔮᐱᔮᐦᑖᑦ ᑐᔅ ᒑ ᒌᐦ ᑯᒋᔥᑎᒥᔮᒡᐦ ᐊᐧᐋᔮᐤᐦ
ᒑᐧᑳᔮᐤ ᐋᐦ ᒥᐧᔫᔮᒡ ᒑ ᒌᐦ ᒦᒋᓈᓂᐧᐃᐧᐃᔮᒡ᙮
ᐊᓐ ᒑᐧᑳᓐ ᐋᑎ ᓂᓂᐦᑖᐅᒋᐦᒡ ᓈᔥᒡ ᐋᐦ
ᐋᔮᒥᐦᒡ ᐋᔨᐧᐃᒄ ᒫᒃ ᐧᐋᐦᒋ ᑯᒋᔥᑖᑦ ᑐᔅ
ᐄᔮᐦᒡ ᐋᐦ ᐄᔑᓈᑯᓂᔮᒡ ᒑᐧᑳᔮᐤ ᒑ ᒌᐦ
ᒦᔥᑯᒋᐱᔮᐦᑖᑭᓂᐧᐃᐧᐃᔮᒡ᙮ ᐋᔨᐧᐃᒄ ᒦᓐ
ᐧᑳᒋᔥᑖᒡ ᒑ ᒌᐦ ᐃᐦᑐᑎᑭᓂᐧᐃᐧᐃᔮᒡ ᐋᑳ
ᒑ ᒌᐦ ᐋᐱᒋᐦᐋᑦ ᐊᐧᐋᓐ ᐅᑖᐹᓈᔅᑯᐦ ᐋᐦ
ᓂᑑᐋᐱᑎᓰᑦ, ᑎᔮᑯᒡ ᒑ ᐱᒧᐦᑖᑦ ᐊᓂᑖᐦ
ᐅᑖᐦᒡ ᑳ ᒌ ᐃᐦᑎᓈᓂᐧᐃᐧᐃᔮᒡ᙮ ᑭᔫᐦ ᔔᐦᒋᒫᐤ
ᐊᐧᐋᔮᐤ ᒑ ᒌᐦ ᐄᑐᐦᑖᔮᒡᐦ ᐊᓂᑖᐦ ᐋᐦ
ᐙᐙᐅᐱᔮᐦᐅᓈᓂᐧᐃᐧᐃᔮᒡ, ᐋᑦ ᑭᔮᐧᐹ ᐋᑳ
ᓈᔥᒡ ᒧᒋᐦᐄᑯᔮᒡᐦ ᓃᔥᑎᒻ᙮ ᒋᓵᓰᐲᐦᒡ ᒫᒃ
ᓈᓈᓂᒌᒻ ᐄᔮᐦᒡ ᐄᔅᐱᔮᐤ ᒑᐧᑳᓐ: ᐊᑎᑎᐤ
ᐱᐹᒧᐦᑖᐧᐃᒡ ᐊᐧᐋᓂᒌ ᐊᓂᑖᐦ ᒫᔅᑭᓈᐦᒡ ᑭᔫᐦ
ᒫᒃ ᐊᓂᑖᐦ ᔫᔫᐤ ᓰᐲᐦᒡ ᓈᐱᓂᔮᒡᐦ ᑭᔫᐦ
ᑭᒐᑭᓵᒫᐧᐃᒡ ᐊᐧᐋᓂᒌ ᐊᓂᑖᐦ ᐋᐦ ᐱᐳᓂᔮᒡ᙮
ᒥᒄ ᒫᒃ ᐋᔥᒄ ᐅᔫ ᐊᓅᐦᒡ ᓂᒥ ᐧᐋᐱᒫᐤ ᑐᔅ
ᐊᐧᐋᔮᐤᐦ ᐋᐦ ᐧᐄᒋᐱᐦᑖᒫᔮᒡᐦ ᐅᑖᒥᔮᐤᐦ᙮

ᐄᓅᔮᒥᐦᐁᐤ ᐁ ᐊᔮᒥᐦᐋᑦ ᐁ ᐧᐋᐧᐄᐦᑕᒧᐧᐋᑦ
ᑖᓐ ᒉ ᐃᔑ ᓇᓈᑲᒋᐦᐄᓯᔮᒡ ᐁ ᔒᐧᐋᑲᒥᐦᐧᑫᔮᒡ᙮
ᐊᓄᐦᒌᔥ ᒫᒃ, ᒥᓯᐧᐁ ᐁ ᑕᐦᑐᑌᐅᓰᓈᓅᒡ
ᒋᓴᓰᐲᐦᒡ ᒌ ᑖᐦᑲᐦᐆᑯᐧᐃᒡ ᐅᔩ ᐋᐦᑯᓯᐧᐃᓂᔩ
ᑲᔦ ᐧᐁᑖᒡ ᒥᐦᒉᑑᒡ ᐁ ᐊᐧᐋᔒᐅᐧᑖᐤ ᐊᐧᐁᓂᒌ
ᐁ ᔒᐧᐋᑲᒥᐦᐧᑫᐧᑖᐤ᙮ ᐧᐄᔪ ᐱᒥᐸᔮᐦᑖᐤ ᐧᓵᔅ
ᐁ ᐧᐋᐸᐦᑎᔫᑲᓅᐧᑖᐤ ᐊᐧᐁᓂᒌ ᒉᒄ ᒦᒋᒥᔩ ᒉ
ᒥᔩᔅᑲᑯᐧᑖᐤ ᑲᔦ ᑯᒋᔥᑕᒧᔦᐤ ᐊᓂᔩ ᒦᒋᒥᔩ᙮
ᓈᔅᒡ ᑖᐧᐯ ᐙᓚᔫᐅᓐ ᐊᓇᐦᐄ ᓇᓈᐦᑰ ᑳ
ᐃᔑᓈᑯᐦᐧᑳᐤᐦ ᒦᒋᒻ ᐁᒌ ᓂᐦᑖᐅᒋᐦᑖᑲᓅᐦᐧᑳᐤ
ᑲᔦ ᐧᐋᐱᒥᓂᒡ, ᒦᓂᔅ ᒥᓯᐧᐁ ᐁ ᐃᔑᓈᑯᐦᐧᑳᐤ
ᐁᒄ ᒫᒃ ᓇᒧᐃ ᐧᐄᐦ ᐅᑎᓇᒻ ᐊᐧᐁᓐ ᐸᔅᒡ
ᐊᓂᔩᐦ ᐁᑳ ᒋᔅᑫᔮᐦᑕᐦᒃ ᒉ ᐧᐄᐦᒋᔥᑕᒧᐧᑫ᙮
ᐁᐅᒄ ᒫᒃ ᐁ ᐃᐦᑎᑦ ᐧᓵᔅ ᐧᐋᐸᐦᑎᔦᐤ ᐊᓂᔩᐦ
ᒦᒋᒻᐦ ᑲᔦ ᑯᒋᔥᑕᒧᔦᐤ ᐁᒄ ᓇᒧᐃ ᐧᐊᓂᐦᑖᐅᒡ
ᐙᓚᔫᔩ᙮ ᐧᐄ ᓇᓈᑲᒋᐦᑖᐤ ᑲᔦ ᐁ ᓰᐦᒋᒫᐧᑖᐤ
ᐊᐧᐁᔩ ᒉᒌ ᐱᒧᐦᑌᔮᒡ ᐃᔅᐱᔥ ᐧᐄ ᒉᒌ
ᐱᒦᐸᔮᔮᒡ ᐅᑖᐹᓂᔩ ᐁ ᓂᑑ ᐋᐸᑎᓯᔮᒡ,
ᐧᐁᔥ ᐁᑯᓐ ᑳᒌ ᐃᐦᑎᐧᑖᐤ ᐊᓂᔦᐦᑳᓈᓂᒡ
ᒋᒧᐙᒥᓅᒡ ᑲᔦ ᒎᐦᑯᒥᓅᐦᒡ ᒨᔥ ᒌ ᐱᒧᐦᑌᐅᒡ᙮
ᓰᐦᒋᒧᐧᐁᐤ ᑲᔦ ᒉᒌ ᓂᑑ ᓴᓵᐅᐧᐃᔮᒡ ᐊᐧᐁᔩᐦ
ᐊᓂᑌ ᐁ ᐃᐦᑕᑯᓂᔮᐧᑳᐤ ᐊᓂᔩ ᒉᐧᑳᔩ ᒉᒌ
ᐋᐸᒋᐦᑖᐧᑖᐤ ᐅᔩ ᒉᒌ ᐃᐦᑎᐧᑖᐤ ᐋᑦ ᑮᐸ
ᓃᔥᑕᒻ ᐁᐧᐄ ᐱᒫᒥᓯᔮᒡ ᔫᐸᒡ ᓰᒃ ᒉᒌ
ᑯᒋᐦᑖᔮᒡ᙮ ᒥᔅᑕᐦᐄ ᓅᑯᓐ ᐊᓂᑕ ᒋᓴᓰᐲᐦᒡ
ᐋᐦᒌᐤᐦ ᐁ ᐊᑎ ᐃᔅᐸᔮᐦᒡ: ᐧᐁᑖᒡ ᒥᐦᒉᑑᒡ
ᐊᐧᐁᓂᒌ ᓇᓈᐦᑰ ᒉᐧᑳᔩ ᐁ ᐃᐦᑑᑕᐦᐧᑳᐤ ᐁᐧᐄ
ᓴᓵᐧᐃᔮᐧᑖᐤ, ᐱᒧᐦᑌᐅᒡ ᑯᑕᑲᒡ ᐁ ᐅᑖᑯᔑᔮᒡ
ᐊᓂᑌ ᔫᐃᔅᑲᓅ ᒫᒃ ᔫᔦᐤ ᓰᐲᐦᒡ, ᑲᔦ ᑯᑕᑲᒡ
ᒋᑳᔅᒣᐦᑌᐅᒡ ᐊᓂᑌ ᓂᑐᐧᐄᓐ ᐁ ᐱᒧᐦᑌᐧᑖᐤ ᐁ
ᐱᐳᓂᔮᒡ᙮ ᐁᔅᒄ ᒥᒄ ᓇᒧᐃ ᐅᒋ ᐧᐋᐸᒣᐤ ᐧᓵᔅ
ᐊᐧᐁᔩ ᒉᒌ ᐱᒥᐸᐦᑖᔮᒡ ᐊᑎᒻ ᐁ ᐅᑖᐱᐦᐋᔮᒡ᙮

leur propre langue, comment gérer la maladie. À l'heure actuelle, toutes les familles de Chisasibi sont directement touchées par le diabète et les personnes nouvellement diagnostiquées sont de plus en plus jeunes. Rose organise des dégustations d'aliments sains. Les fruits et légumes sont si chers dans le Nord que les gens ne veulent pas dépenser d'argent pour en acheter de nouveaux qu'ils n'aimeraient peut-être pas. Aussi, Rose trouve des moyens de leur faire goûter de nouveaux aliments sans qu'ils aient à dépenser tout cet argent. Elle organise aussi des journées « Laissez-votre-voiture-à-la-maison » pour que les gens puissent essayer de faire de l'exercice en rendant au travail, comme le faisaient leurs grands-parents. Et elle encourage les gens à essayer le centre de conditionnement physique, même si c'est un peu intimidant au début. Chisasibi connaît à nouveau de grands changements : les gens font plus d'exercice, marchent dehors le long de l'autoroute ou de la rivière pendant les longues soirées d'été, ou font de la raquette dans les grands espaces en hiver. Jusqu'à présent, toutefois, Rose n'a vu personne courir à côté d'un attelage de chiens.

disease. By now, every Chisasibi family is directly affected by diabetes and the newly diagnosed are getting younger and younger. Rose organizes healthy-food tastings. Vegetables and fruits are so expensive in the North that people don't want to spend money on new ones they might not like, so Rose finds ways to let them taste new foods without having to pay all that money. She also organizes Leave-Your-Vehicle-At-Home days for people to try exercising as a way of getting to work, as their grandparents once did. And she encourages people to try the fitness centre, even if it is a little intimidating at first. Chisasibi is seeing big changes again: people are exercising more, walking outside along the highway or the river in the long summer evenings, or snowshoeing across the open spaces in winter. So far, though, Rose hasn't seen anyone running alongside a dog team.

ᐧᒫᐦᒡ ᒫᒃ ᐊᓂᔮᐦ ᒥᓯᐧᐋ ᐋᔑ ᒋᔅᑯᑎᒧᐧᐋᑦ ᐊᐧᐋᔭᐤᐦ ᐧᐄᔭ ᑭᔮᐦ ᒍᔅ ᒋᑭ ᓈᓈᑭᒋᐦᑖᐤ ᐊᓂᔮ ᐋᐦ ᔖᑳᐅᐱᔭᑦ ᐋᔑᑯᒥᒌᔑᑳᐤᐦ᙮ ᐅᑎᓂᒻ ᐅᓂᑎᐦᑯᔭᓂᒻᐦ ᑭᔮᐦ ᓂᑑᑎᐹᔭᐦᑎᒻ ᐅᒥᐦᒄ ᐋᔅᐱᔭᔭᐤ᙮ ᑯᒋᔅᑖᐤ ᓂᓈᐦᑭᐤ ᐋᐦ ᐄᔑᓈᑯᓂᔭᐤ ᒦᒋᒥᔭᐤ ᒑ ᓂᐦᐄᔥᑳᑯᑦ ᐅᔮᐦᒡ᙮ ᐋᔦᐧᐃᒄ ᓈᔥᒡ ᒑ ᐧᐄᐦ ᓈᑭᑎᐧᐋᔭᑎᐦᒃ ᐋᑳ ᓈᔥᒡ ᒑ ᒌᐦ ᒫᑯᔥᑳᑯᑦ ᒑᐧᑳᔭᐤ ᐋᐦ ᐄᔅᐱᔭᔭᐤ = ᐋᐅᒄ ᐆ ᓈᔥᒡ ᐧᐋᒋᐦᐄᐧᐋᐱᔭᐤ ᒑ ᒌᐦ ᐄᔅᑯᐱᐦᑖᒥᑭᓂᓂᔭᐤ ᐊᐧᐋᓐ ᐅᔖᑲᒻ᙮ ᓈᔥᑖᐧᐹᐦ ᐧᐄᒋᐦᐄᐧᐋᐤ ᑯᐃᔅᒄ ᐋᐦ ᔮᔮᐦᓂᐧᐃᐤ ᑭᔮᐦ ᒥᒄ ᐋᐦ ᐊᔭᒥᐦᒋᑳᓂᐧᐃᐤ, ᐋᐦ ᐊᔭᒥᐦᑖᑭᓂᐧᐃᐤ ᑭᔭᐧᐹ ᒥᓯᓂᐦᐄᑭᓐ᙮ ᓈᑖᐦ ᒫᒃ ᐄᔑ ᐅᑖᐦᒡ ᐊᓂᔮ ᐋᐦ ᒌᐦ ᒥᓂᐦᐧᑳᔭᐦᒡ ᐅᓈᐹᒻᐦ ᐋᑯᑎᐦ ᓈᔥᒡ ᓂᒥ ᐅᐦᒋ ᒥᔦᑑᑖᑯᐧᐋᐤ, ᒥᒄ ᒫᒃ ᐊᓅᐦᒡ ᐋᑎᐧᐄ ᔖᔥ ᓂᒥ ᒥᓂᐦᐧᑳᔭᐤᐦ᙮ ᐅᔮ ᒫᒃ ᐊᓅᐦᒡ ᐊᓂᔮ ᐅᑎᐧᐋᔑᔒᒻᐦ ᑭᔮᐦ ᐅᔑᔑᒥᔥᐦ ᐋᔦᐧᐃᑯᓐᐦ ᓈᔥᒡ ᐃᔮᔭᒫᔭᐦᑎᒥᐦᐄᑯᑦ, ᐋᔅᑭᐤ ᐋᐦ ᑭᓂᐧᐋᔭᐦᑎᔮᑭᓂᐧᐃᑦ ᐊᓂᔮᐦ ᐅᔑᔑᒥᔥᐦ᙮ ᑖᐹ ᐧᐋᐦᑎᓂᔭᐤ ᐊᓂᔮ ᐊᐧᐋᓐ ᐋᐦ ᐅᑎᐦᑎᐦᐅᑯᑦ ᐋᑳ ᔖᔥ ᐄᔥᐱᔑ ᐅᔅᒋᓃᒌᑦ ᑳᔥᐱᔥ ᐅᔅᒋᓃᒌᑦ ᒍᔅ ᐋᔥᒄ ᐋᐦ ᒌᐦ ᐧᐄᒑᐧᐋᑦ ᒫᓐᐦ ᐅᒧᔔᒻᐦ ᐊᑎᒻᐦ ᐋᐦ ᐋᐱᒋᐦᐋᒡ᙮

ᐋᑯᐦ ᐋᑎᑯᑦ ᐅᓈᐹᒻᐦ, “ᒍᔅ ᒋᓂᔥᑎᐧᐃᓈᑯᓯᓐ ᐋᐦ ᐅᑎᐦᒋᐱᔭᐤ ᒑ ᐱᐹᒧᐦᑖᔭᐦᒄ᙮”

ᒉᔑᑯᒻ ᒌᔑᑳᐤ ᓇᓈᑲᒋᐦᐄᔦ ᑲᔦ ᐧᐄᔭ ᐧᑫᔅ ᐁ ᔩᐧᐋᑲᒥᐦᐧᑫᑦ ᒧᐧᐁᐦᒡ ᐁ ᐃᐦᑎᔭᐤ ᐊᓂᔦᐦ ᑳ ᒋᔅᑯᑕᒧᐧᐋᑦ ᒉ ᐃᔑ ᑲᓇᐧᐁᔭᒥᓯᔭᐤ᙮ ᐅᑎᓇᒻ ᐅᓂᑐᐦᑯᐄᓂᒻᐦ ᑲᔦ ᓂᑑ ᒋᔅᒉᔭᐦᑕᒻ ᐅᒥᐦᒄ ᑖᓂᑕ ᐁ ᐃᐦᑕᑯᓂᔭᐤ᙮ ᓇᓈᐦᑰ ᒦᒋᒻ ᐁᒌ ᓂᐦᑖᐅᒋᐦᑖᑲᓅᔭᐧᑳᐤ ᑲᔦ ᑳ ᐸᐦᐧᑫᔑᑲᓅᓂᔭᐧᑳᐤ ᒦᒎ ᒥᔅᑕᐦᐄ ᐁ ᐃᐦᑕᑯᓂᔭᐤ ᐊᓂᑕ ᒉᐧᑳᔦ ᐁ ᒥᔦᔅᑲᒉᒪᑲᓂᔭᐤ᙮ ᐃᔑᓈᑯᓂᔦ ᑲᔦ ᒉᒌ ᓇᓈᑲᒋᐦᑖᑦ ᐁᑳ ᓈᔅᒡ ᒉᒌ ᒥᑯᔥᑳᑌᔭᐦᑕᒥᐦᐄᑯᑦ ᒉᐧᑳᔦ = ᐁᐅᑰ ᐯᔭᒄ ᒉᐧᑳᓐ ᐁ ᐃᐦᑑᑖᒉᒪᑲᐦᒡ ᒉᒌ ᐃᔅᐧᑳᐦᒋᐸᔭᓂᔭᐤ ᐊᐧᐁᓐ ᐁ ᔖᑳᐅᐸᔭᑦ᙮ ᐊᐧᐁᓐ ᑳ ᐋᔭᒉᔭᐦᑕᒥᐦᐄᑯᑦ ᒉᐧᑳᔦ ᒋᑲ ᐧᐄᒋᐦᐄᑰ ᒉᒌ ᐊᔭᐧᐁᔩᑦ ᐧᐁᐃᐱᔅᒌᔥ ᑯᑕᒋᔦ ᒉᐧᑳᔦ ᒉᒌ ᐃᐦᑑᑕᐦᒃ ᒧᐧᐁᐦᒡ ᒪᓯᓇᐦᐄᑲᓂᔦ ᐊᔭᒥᐦᑖᑦ ᒫᒃ ᒥᒄ ᐃᔅᑯᑖᒧᑦ ᑲᔦ ᓃᐦᑕᑖᒧᑦ ᐁᑯᓐ ᒉᒌ ᐃᐦᑎᑦ᙮ ᐧᐁᔅᑲᒡ ᐊᓂᑌ ᐃᔑ ᐅᑖᐦᒡ, ᓈᔅᒡ ᒌ ᐋᔭᒉᔭᐦᑕᒥᐦᐄᑰ ᐅᓈᐯᒻ ᐁ ᒥᓂᐦᐧᑫᔭᐤ ᒥᒄ ᒫᒃ ᔮᔅ ᒥᐦᒉᑐᐱᐳᓐᐦ ᑳ ᐴᓂᔭᐤ ᐁ ᒥᓂᐦᐧᑫᔭᐤ᙮ ᐃᐦᑖᔦ ᐅᑕᐧᐋᔒᒧᐧᐋᐤᐦ ᑲᔦ ᐅᔑᒧᐧᐋᐤᐦ ᐁ ᐸᐹᒉᔭᒫᑦ ᐧᑫᔅ ᐋᔅᑰ ᒫᒃ ᑲᓇᐧᐁᔭᒉᐤ ᐸᔅᒡ ᐊᓂᔦᐦ ᐅᔑᒻᐦ ᐊᓂᑕ ᒉᐧᑳᒡ ᐁᑳ ᒌ ᐋᔮᐅᑯᔭᒡ ᐅᓃᒋᐦᐄᑯᔦᐦ᙮ ᐋᔭᒥᐦᐄᑰ ᑲᔦ ᐧᐄ ᒥᑯᔥᑳᑌᔭᐦᑕᒻ ᓂᔮᓂᑯᑌᐦᒡ ᔮᔅ ᑮᐹ ᐁ ᐊᑎ ᒋᒐᐃᓅᔑᑦ ᐁᑳ ᐃᔑᓈᑯᓯᑦ ᐁᔅᒄ ᐁᒌ ᐊᐧᐋᔒᐅᑦ ᐅᒧᔖᒻ ᐅᑖᐹᓈᔅᑯᔭᐤ ᑳᒌᐦ ᑌᐦᑕᐱᑦ ᐁ ᐅᑖᐹᑎᑯᑦ ᐊᑎᒻᐦ᙮

ᐄᑎᑰ ᒫᓐᐦ ᐅᓈᐯᓐ, “ᐧᑫᔦ, ᓂᒋᔅᒉᔭᐦᑌᓐ ᐁ ᑲᓇᐧᐋᐸᐦᑕᒫᓐ ᒋᑖᔅᑕᒥᐦᒄ, ᒋᐹ ᒥᐧᔮᔖ ᓂᑑ ᐸᐹᒧᐦᑌᔭᐦᒄ᙮”

Comme tous les gens à qui elle enseigne, Rose doit travailler sur son propre diabète tous les jours. Elle prend ses pilules et teste son taux de sucre dans le sang. Elle fait des expériences avec des légumes et cuisine avec des grains entiers et des aliments à forte teneur en fibres. Elle doit faire particulièrement attention au stress – c'est la seule chose qui fait augmenter son taux de glycémie très rapidement. Parfois, se calmer se résume à prendre quelques grandes respirations ou à lire un bon livre. Il y a quelques années, l'alcoolisme de son mari était ce qui faisait monter son anxiété, mais il ne boit plus depuis des années. Ces jours-ci, Rose s'inquiète pour ses enfants et ses petits-enfants et s'occupe aussi de certains de ses petits-enfants les jours où ils sont négligés. Cela fait beaucoup de travail et d'anxiété pour une personne qui n'est plus assez jeune pour s'asseoir sur le traîneau à chiens de son grand-père.

Like all the people she teaches, Rose has to work at her own diabetes every day. She takes her pills and tests her blood sugar. She experiments with vegetables and cooks with whole grains and high fibre. She has to be especially careful about stress – it's the one thing drives up her blood sugar levels very quickly. Sometimes calming down is as easy as taking a few deep breaths or reading a good book. Years ago, her husband's drinking was what drove up her anxiety, but he hasn't had a drink in years. These days, Rose worries for her kids and grandkids and also looks after some of her grandkids on the days they're neglected. It gets to be a lot of work and anxiety for someone no longer young enough to sit on her grandfather's dogsled.

Alors son mari lui dit : « Oh Rosie. Je peux le voir sur ton visage, il est temps d'aller prendre une marche ».

Then her husband says, "Oh Rosie. I can see on your face – it's time to go for a walk."

ᓈᐦᒋᓈᑯᒡ ᑮᔮᐦ ᓈᐦᒋᓈᑯᓈᒡ ᐅᔑᔑᒥᔑᐙᐤᐦ
ᐋᐦ ᒌᓲᐦᐅᒡ ᐊᓂᔮ ᑭᔭᐿ ᓈᔥᒡ ᐋᐦ ᑎᐦᑳᔮᔭᒡ
ᓈᑖᐦ ᒫᐢᑭᓈᐦᐦᒡ ᐋᑎ ᐱᐹᒧᐦᑖᒡ ᐊᓂᑖᐦ ᒑ ᒌᐦ
ᒫᑎᐙᔭᒡᐦ ᐅᔑᔑᒥᔑᐙᐤᐦ ᑰᓂᐦᐦᒡ᙮

ᐁᒄ ᑮᐹ ᒉ ᐳᐢᒋᔥᑲᐦᒁᐤ ᐅᒪᐢᒋᓯᓇᐙᐤ
ᑲᔦ ᐐᔮᐢᐱᑖᑣᐤ ᐅᔑᒧᐙᐤᐦ ᐁ ᑕᐦᑳᔮᔭᒡ
ᐐᐐᑎᒥᐦᐦᒡ ᐁᒄ ᒉ ᒋᐢᑐᐦᑌᑣᐤ ᓀᑌ
ᐅᑖᐹᓂᒉᐢᑲᓈᐦᐦᒡ ᒉ ᓂᑑ ᐱᒧᐦᑌᑣᐤ᙮ ᐁ
ᒥᔩᒌᐃᔑᑳᔑᔭᒡ ᑲᔦ ᐁ ᒨᒋᑲᐦᑖᔭᒡ ᐅᔑᒧᐙᐤ
ᑰᓐ ᐁ ᑖᐦᑕᐦᒋᔥᑯᐙᑣᐤ ᐊᓂᔩ ᐁ ᐱᒧᐦᑌᑣᐤ᙮

Et ils attachent leurs bottes et emmitouflent les petits-enfants pour les protéger du froid, et partent pour une longue promenade au bord de la route où le soleil scintille sur les congères et où les petits-enfants font voler la neige autour d’eux.

And they tie on their boots and swaddle the grandkids against the cold and head out for a long walk by the highway where the sun glints off the snowdrifts and the grandkids kick up snow around them.

Syllabic Chart
Tableau de caractères syllabiques

ᐄᔨᔨᐅᔥᑖᐤ

ᐄᓅᔥᑌᐤ

ᐁ e		ᐃ i	ᐄ ii	ᐅ u	ᐆ uu	ᐊ a	ᐋ aa		ᐤ u	ᐦ h
	ᐌ we	ᐎ wi	ᐐ wii	ᐒ wu	ᐔ wuu	ᐗ wa		ᐙ waa		
ᐯ pe	ᐺ pwe	ᐱ pi	ᐲ pii	ᐳ pu	ᐴ puu	ᐸ pa	ᐹ paa	ᑆ pwaa	ᑉ p	
ᑌ te	ᑗ twe	ᑎ ti	ᑏ tii	ᑐ tu	ᑑ tuu	ᑕ ta	ᑖ taa	ᑣ twaa	ᑦ t	
ᑫ ke	ᑵ kwe	ᑭ ki	ᑮ kii	ᑯ ku	ᑰ kuu	ᑲ ka	ᑳ kaa	ᒁ kwaa	ᒃ k	ᒄ kw
ᒉ che	ᒒ chwe	ᒋ chi	ᒌ chii	ᒍ chu	ᒎ chuu	ᒐ cha	ᒑ chaa	ᒞ chwaa	ᒡ ch	
ᒣ me	ᒬ mwe	ᒥ mi	ᒦ mii	ᒧ mu	ᒨ muu	ᒪ ma	ᒫ maa	ᒸ mwaa	ᒻ m	ᒼ mw
ᓀ ne	ᓊ nwe	ᓂ ni	ᓃ nii	ᓄ nu	ᓅ nuu	ᓇ na	ᓈ naa	ᓎ nwaa	ᓐ n	
ᓓ le	ᓜ lwe	ᓕ li	ᓖ lii	ᓗ lu	ᓘ luu	ᓚ la	ᓛ laa	ᓨ lwaa	ᓪ l	
ᓭ se	ᓶ swe	ᓯ si	ᓰ sii	ᓱ su	ᓲ suu	ᓴ sa	ᓵ saa	ᔂ swaa	ᔅ s	
ᔐ she	ᔗ shwe	ᔑ shi	ᔒ shii	ᔓ shu	ᔔ shuu	ᔕ sha	ᔖ shaa	ᔣ shwaa	ᔥ sh	
ᔦ ye	ᔯ ywe	ᔨ yi	ᔩ yii	ᔪ yu	ᔫ yuu	ᔭ ya	ᔮ yaa	ᔻ ywaa	ᔾ y	
ᕃ re	ᐧᕃ rwe	ᕆ ri	ᕇ rii	ᕈ ru	ᕉ ruu	ᕋ ra	ᕌ raa	ᕍ rwaa	ᕐ r	
ᕓ ve	ᐧᕓ vwe	ᕕ vi	ᕖ vii	ᕗ vu	ᕘ vuu	ᕙ va	ᕚ vaa	ᕛ vwaa	ᕝ v/f/ph	
ᕞ the	ᐧᕞ thwe	ᕠ thi	ᕡ thii	ᕢ thu	ᕣ thuu	ᕤ tha	ᕥ thaa	ᕦ thwaa	ᕪ th	